Kindest rega[illegible]

Rabbi [illegible]

MY LIFE AS A CHAPLAIN

The Mount Sinai Medical Center

on the occasion of his retirement

Honors

Rabbi Dr. Charles A. Spirn
Head Chaplain
1979-1998

for his distinguished service

Your compassionate spiritual leadership and guidance, creative initiatives, and exemplary dedication to our patients, families, and staff are deeply appreciated and will be long remembered.

March 31, 1998
New York, New York

MY LIFE AS A CHAPLAIN

How a Hospital Chaplain Helps Patients

by

Charles A. Spirn

SHENGOLD BOOKS

ISBN: 0-88400-209-8
Library of Congress Catalog Card Number: 00 132751

Published by Shengold
Rockville, MD

First Edition 2000

Dedicated

to my dear wife, Dr. Regina Spirn
to my dear children and their spouses
Batya and Ari Jerenberg
Rabbi Nahum and Rebecca Spirn
and to our dear grandchildren.

CONTENTS

RECOMMENDATION FOR A PRESIDENTIAL SERVICE AWARD 1994

A Presidential Service Award is given yearly by the hospital to two outstanding employees of The Mount Sinai Medical Center, based on three criteria of excellence. The following was submitted by a Mount Sinai physician nominating Rabbi Spirn for the award as the rationale for his choice:

Criterion 1: Provided excellent service, of highest merit:

There was no chaplaincy department before Rabbi Spirn's arrival. He established a chaplaincy program and gave it a content far exceeding most others. He also heads a team of multi-faith chaplains.

Since his arrival, there has been a very great change in the way Jewish patients, and in a way all patients, feel that their needs are taken care of at our hospital.

Rabbi Spirn visits weekly *all* Jewish patients, 40 percent of total patient population (1,122) plus extra visits. Since the turnover in my departments, Maternity and Pediatrics, is high, he visits them twice a week instead of once.

He has provided counsel and assistance to patients and their families as well as to staff in a variety of realms, from personal and family problems to resourcefully and wisely finding ways of getting patients to cooperate with necessary procedures.

Going beyond the call of duty is natural to him. He shuns no overwork and frequently stays overtime. He takes initiative in getting things done, and done well. He speaks five languages, which enables him to communicate directly with people of non-English backgrounds.

He is often a confidant to patients and staff and is very efficient and profoundly humane, relating to patients with care and empathy. When others are upset by crisis, like death, he remains calm and thoughtful and offers soothing prayers and guidance.

Scores of letters of thanks come in to Mr. Barry Freedman, director, [now executive vice president] and to the Rabbi himself, commenting on the help and support they have received.

Criterion 2: Demonstrated major contributions and leadership to patients and/or staff, and to the mission and goals of The Mount Sinai Medical Center:

Due to his initiative, dedication, and persuasion, he inaugurated seventeen extra projects to make patients feel at ease here, including very religious patients.

Our kitchen was nonkosher from 1866. In 1990, Rabbi Spirn's initiative led to establishing a kosher kitchen and cafeteria. The present beautiful Jewish chapel was created due to his efforts.

His religious services are thoroughly planned and uplifting to patients. He also fosters and participates in weekday afternoon services for staff and visitors.

He enhances celebration of all Jewish holidays in the hospital. Two hundred patients and staff attend his Passover *Seder*, which he holds at night, after which, at 10:30 P.M., he conducts his home *Seder*.

He increases beauty and inspiration in functions he performs, regularly adding a concert by an outside artist or a choir to make Hanukkah enjoyable for patients, families and staff. He is here *six days a week*, including Saturdays.

On High Holy Days, he transforms a conglomerate audience into a unified congregation, enabling people to feel they have understood the service, its meaning and its relevant message for today. Sabbath and holiday electric candelabra were built into walls at bedsides at his suggestion.

He gives orientation and instructs chaplains about work in our hospital and is the liaison between hospital and representatives of all religious faiths.

At outside meetings, he speaks about Mount Sinai and publishes articles in Anglo-Jewish and Yiddish weeklies, thus promoting our hospital. He writes exceedingly well.

Criterion 3: Consistently receives above average performance appraisals:

He plans projects well ahead of time and works out all details meticulously.

His performance has been evaluated as "Superior" by his supervisor of more than fourteen years, Ms. Sylvia M. Barker, and Dr. Gail Kuhn Weissman, vice president of nursing, to which chaplaincy was attached till now.

Summary:

Rabbi Spirn is a unique combination of qualities: ordination from Yeshiva University and a Ph.D. in French Literature from Columbia University. He is a man of religion with a rich background in the humanities and a clinically certified chaplain (certified by the National Association of Jewish Chaplains) – all that is of inestimable import to our hospital. We are indeed fortunate to have a man of his caliber on our staff.

COMMENTS BY ADMINISTRATION

The Mount Sinai Medical Center
Office of the Chairman

The Mount Sinai Hospital
Mount Sinai School of Medicine

One Gustave L. Levy Place
New York, NY 10029-6574

November 15, 1995

Rabbi Charles Spirn
Box 1036
Mount Sinai Medical Center
1 Gustave Levy Place
New York, NY 10029

Dear Rabbi Spirn:

This is just a note to thank you for sending along your Annual Report of the Chaplaincy Department. It is inspiring to read about how you respond in such a humane and comprehensive fashion to the spiritual needs of the Mount Sinai family.

Judith and I derive great satisfaction in the knowledge of the extensive use of the Peck Chapel.

I also want to thank you for your kind and generous reference to my new responsibilities with the Boards of Mount Sinai Medical Center.

Judith joins me in kind regards to you.

Sincerely,
Stephen M. Peck
Chairman, Boards of Trustees
The Mount Sinai Medical Center

Rabbi Charles A. Spirn
Head Chaplain
The Mount Sinai Medical Center
One Gustave Levy Place
New York, NY 10029

November 17, 1982

Dear Rabbi Spirn:

I am putting in writing what Reba has already told you – that I found your latest report very impressive. We try very hard to anticipate the needs of our patients. Then, after I've read your report, I realize how far-reaching human needs can be and how important the Chaplain's role can be.

You are an important factor in our ability to give superior patient care, and we are grateful to you.

Sincerely,

Thomas C. Chalmers, M.D.
President and Dean
The Mount Sinai Hospital
and School of Medicine

October 17, 1988

Dear Rabbi Spirn:

Thank you very much for sending me the Annual Report of your Chaplaincy activities. I have read the document with great interest and am impressed by the scope of efforts that you have initiated. I have heard from several faculty of the outstanding contributions that you are making to Mount Sinai. With the opening of our new hospital, and the availability of a new, proper synagogue, I am sure that your efforts will be even further enhanced.

You are an important part of the overall mission of this institution to provide the highest quality health care services. Thank you for your efforts.

Warmest regards,
John W. Rowe, M.D.
President
The Mount Sinai Medical Center

February 25, 1998

Dear Rabbi Spirn:

It is hard to realize that you are about to retire as Head Chaplain here at Mount Sinai. I know, from the many warm and complimentary letters you have shared with me over the years and the comments others have made to our office, that your presence has had a significant and positive impact on our patients and their families.

I join with my colleagues in wishing you and your wife a fulfilling new life in retirement with our heartfelt thanks for your many years of service dedicated to helping others.

Sincerely,
Barry R. Freedman
Executive Vice President

January 5, 1990

Dear Rabbi Spirn:

You have touched every walk of life... Your mark has been left on so many in dire need, whether it be someone in need of religion, or someone in need of a friend...My hope is for your continued good health, so that your work can go on ad infinitum.

You give to the people you come into contact with the will to survive, and it is so much appreciated. You have really been an inspiration and the office of Religious Affairs has blossomed under your tutelage.

Sincerely,
Gail Kuhn-Weissman, Ed.D., RN, FAAN
Vice President, Nursing

December 4, 1997

Rabbi Charles A. Spirn, Ph.D.
Head Chaplain
The Mount Sinai Medical Center

Dear Rabbi Spirn,

I wish to thank you for sending me a copy of the eighteenth anniversary issue of the Annual Report of the Chaplaincy Department. I read it with great pleasure. It is a comprehensive, often moving, compendium of the many essential functions of the Chaplaincy Department. You have touched on all these aspects in a most impressive way as you describe the traditional services, the counseling role, and the educational and collaborative contributions made by the department. Again, thank you, and congratulations on this report which reflects, as you so well put it, "a well-run, effective, caring and compassionate chaplaincy corps".

Yours truly,
Susan Blumenfield, D.S.W.
Director, Social Work
Services
Supervisor of Chaplaincy

Dear Rabbi Spirn,

I know that your years of service and dedication to Mt. Sinai were well organized and greatly appreciated by both staff, patients, and families and that you had a tremendous impact on many of the people that you worked with. I hope that you and your family are enjoying this time together.

I was happy to have had the pleasure of working with you!
Wishing you all the best – A happy and healthy New Year!

Fondly,
Loren Susser, C.S.W.
Department of Social Work
Recent Administrator of Chaplaincy

EXCERPTS FROM FAREWELL RECEPTION TALK BY ASSOCIATE DIRECTOR, NURSING AFFAIRS

Rabbi Spirn's credentials were superior, his ideas for implementing the program and his apparent dedication to his calling as a rabbi were noteworthy. I was captivated by the potential I perceived for our fledgling program under this man's direction. And so in due time, I, along with others on the interviewing team, particularly Dr. Gary Rosenberg, vice president, Human Resources, recommended Rabbi Spirn for the position...Yearly for eighteen years, Rabbi Spirn has published an annual report of the activities and growth of the program. Through this report and his availability to speak at a variety of conferences and meetings, he has brought the program to the attention of other institutions, leaders, and organizations, so that some of its features have been duplicated across the land...

His Annual Reports were always well presented, interesting and challenging. They revealed the vitality of his program, as well as himself.

His job performance was consistently rated as "Superior". Rabbi Spirn is a dedicated practitioner of his profession...As a counselor for the patients, the staff, the community, and as an interpreter of Jewish Religious Laws, he has no peer. The frequently received letters of appreciation for kindness done, for pastoral services provided, for religious services conducted, attest to the role he plays so very well.

Rabbi Spirn, you will be missed by many – we who are gathered here today wish you the very best of retirement years ahead. You can leave here with the knowledge that you have been instrumental in setting the course of the Chaplaincy Program of The Mount Sinai Medical Center for years to come.

Sylvia M. Barker, RN, MA, CNAA
Fourteen-Year Supervisor of Chaplaincy
March 31, 1998

1: INTRODUCTION

How did the profession of hospital chaplain arise? How did a rabbi become a permanent member of a hospital team composed primarily of physicians, nurses, and social workers?

With the enormous progress in medicine, the hopes for recovery after hospitalization have risen very high. Yet, let us follow a patient as he checks into a hospital – a person who until now has been relatively healthy, active, and independent in his profession, perhaps highly recognized in society, now suddenly isolated and lonely, worried about facing a serious, even life-threatening, illness. In short, the patient faces a crisis. What is more, in a hospital room, a tag is attached to his wrist, and he is referred to by his room and bed number, like "K-831-B," and by the nature of his illness, such as "He is a cardiac patient." Then the impersonal staff comes to him: doctors, residents, medical students, nurses, dieticians, social workers, therapists, and others.

To overcome this depersonalization and assist in overcoming the crisis, the concept of holistic medicine came to the fore, to teach us that we ought to treat the whole person and not limit ourselves to the disease alone. It stresses that we have here a human personality with spiritual and personal dimensions. We must see the patient not only as a medical "case" but also as a man or woman endowed with dignity, what the Bible calls a being created in the image of God (in Hebrew: *Tzelem Elokim*). The holistic concept is relatively new to Western society. To the Jew, however, the concept is ancient and – what is more important – it is affirmed and imprinted on our consciousness three times daily in our weekday silent prayers called *Shemonay Esray*, recited by the worshipper morning, late afternoon, and evening. Included in this three-time weekday prayer is a supplication for good health in which we affirm that God is *both* a Competent and a Compassionate Healer (*Rofay Neemon Verachamon*). And so, in *Imitatio Dei*, in imitating the Divine Healer, the human physician, too, must be *Neemon*, competent in diagnosing and treating illness, and also *Rachamon*, compassionate to the person he treats.

In accordance with the modern holistic approach to medicine, hospitals have begun to add full-time chaplains to their staff. In Jewish hospitals, each chaplain must be an ordained rabbi and certified as meeting standards of professional competence in Chaplaincy. That means that to him, the patient is not a bed number or a medical case, but primarily a person, a human being, endowed with a Divine soul and dignity, and the chaplain relates to him on that level.

Role of Religion in the Healing Process

Religion has a tremendous value in itself – religious people know that. In a talk delivered to Mount Sinai staff on February 23, 1981, I mentioned some ideas culled from my readings on the role of religion in human life.

Victor Hugo, the great French poet and novelist, remarked about himself that the weaker the body becomes, the stronger waxes one's spirit. It is understood that religious people will cling to religion to the very end of their lives. It is also the experience of clergymen that people who were exposed to religion in their youth will have a strong urge to return to it in their older age, and certainly at a time when life is ebbing away from them, even though religion was minimal or diluted during their active adult years. They feel the need to end their earthly pilgrimage as they had begun it: within the framework of religion. This is a kind of returning to one's roots. However, it has also been my experience and that of others that people nominally irreligious turn to religion at crucial points in their lives and, sure enough, at the end of life. The hospital chaplain's role will then be more far-reaching than what may have been assumed.

The hospital chaplain can therefore exclude no one a priori from his ministrations. The needs will vary from patient to patient, and the chaplain will have to evaluate those spiritual needs and seek to meet them. In these ministrations, the chaplain's role is viewed as that of a representative or symbol of a specific faith-community. However, lest it be overlooked, let us stress that the personal qualities of the chaplain – his love for people, his empathy, his warmth, his concern, and his dedication – will also determine to a significant extent his rapport with patient and family and the effectiveness of his ministrations.

Basically, the hospital chaplain will fulfill three roles:

- Supportive role: through a warm, personal rapport with patient and family, the chaplain will endeavor to strengthen them spiritually and psychologically. He will be an attentive listener and a wise counselor. He will tend to diminish prevailing guilt and show the road to reconciliation and peace of mind and peace of soul.

- Inspirational role: through religious services, through readings of sacred writings and appropriate sermons, through religious practices and rituals, festivals, and ceremonies.
- Guiding role: the patient may seek guidance in family problems and relationship with his children and with his community. Not to be overlooked is the fact that the regular presence of the chaplain often stimulates patient and family to probe into metaphysical questions that lie just beneath the surface. The person may also wish to discuss confidential matters that are on his mind and which, he feels, he can discuss and reveal to a clergyman. It is hoped that the patient and family will take home the inspiration and a degree of peace of mind acquired at the hospital.

What I wish to call attention to is that religion also gives its adherents many ancillary or "fringe" benefits. Thus while pain is not less painful for religious patients, the fact remains that religious people find great support in their faith in God. Daily religious practices, such as praying three times a day, learning, observing commandments, going to sleep at night saying: "The Lord is with me. I shall not be afraid," getting up in the morning and thanking God "for having restored my soul within me, for great is Your faithfulness, Your trustworthiness," these and scores of daily prayer-contacts with Divinity, all have a stabilizing effect on the patient and keep him on an even keel. The fact that the Jewish religion has a structured lifestyle provides extra sources of support to the religious patient. Moreover, by using daily instruments of religion, we not only increase our faith but, lo and behold, we also increase our will to live and our will to recover – and that clearly helps the physician in the healing of the patient. Physicians and psychiatrists know that, and, thus, they value the chaplain's role as a member of the healing team. They often initiate a call to the chaplain to ask for his help in instilling the will to live in a patient or to help him find peace of mind and peace of soul. To sum up: Faith is an asset not only from the religious viewpoint but from the medical viewpoint as well. And, yes, chaplains do offer religious literature to patients of their faith, in the form of prayer pamphlets for daily use and others explaining holidays and their message. It stands to reason that hospitals should foster and not interfere with patients' religious needs, which support him spiritually and emotionally. As for those who consider themselves not religious, they too usually appreciate the ministrations of the chaplain if he knows how to approach them, how to respond to their personal and religious problems and how to move them a little closer to God.

A Brief History of the Mount Sinai Medical Center

The Mount Sinai Hospital was founded in 1852 at 138 West 28th Street under the name of Jews' Hospital by Sampson Simson, an observant religious Jew. The hospital was kosher and had a synagogue. Mr. Simson, a graduate of Columbia College, was the first Jewish lawyer to pass the New York bar examination. In 1852, at the age of seventy-two, he convinced his friends who were prominent in the Spanish-Portuguese Synagogue, called Shearith Israel, the oldest synagogue in the city, to help him plan the Jews' Hospital, referred to in Hebrew as *Bet Cholim*. In 1866, the hospital changed its name to Mount Sinai Hospital, became non-sectarian, and *kashruth* was abandoned. It moved to Lexington Avenue and 66th Street and later, in 1904, to still larger quarters at 100th Street and 5th Avenue where it is located at present. At that location, the hospital transformed its synagogue into a workshop. The School of Medicine opened in 1963, so that Mount Sinai became a teaching hospital as well. Mount Sinai is considered a most prestigious medical center, and many "medical firsts" were discovered by its staff. At the same time, it takes pride in being the flagship of Jewish hospitals in this country and highly renowned throughout the world.

My Ministry at Mount Sinai

I was the first head chaplain of The Mount Sinai Medical Center where I served close to twenty years. Prior to that, I served twenty-eight years as a pulpit rabbi, having received my ordination from Yeshiva University. I am also the recipient of a Ph.D. in French Literature from Columbia University. It was only in 1979 that this, one of the major medical centers in the country, recognized the need to have a rabbi as a permanent, full-time member of its staff. This came about in principle through the influence of the new concept of holistic medicine. Practically, it was made possible by a grant from the Federation of Jewish Philanthropies, obtained by the activist and indefatigable director of its Religious Department, Rabbi Isaac N. Trainin, and the prompting and recommendation of the New York Board of Rabbis, particularly of its gentle and effective executive director, Rabbi Paul L. Hait, under the aegis of whose chaplaincy commission we functioned. In addition, I was recommended for this position by Mr. Victor B. Geller, Dean, and Rabbi Herschel Schacter, Director, of the Division of Community Services of Yeshiva University.

I began my duties as head chaplain in mid-October 1979. Upon assuming my duties, I established a general rule that I visit every Jewish patient at least once a week. Those daily visits, done in accordance with the official list provided by the hospital's Computer Center, constituted the core of my work five days a week. I also led services on Saturdays and holidays and did some extra visiting of patients at the conclusion of our religious services.

To give the reader some conception of the time of the visits, we must keep in mind that Mount Sinai had a total of 1,122 beds. The largest single religious group among our patients was the Jewish group, which comprised 40 percent of the total number of patients, or 450–500 patients. I visited all our pavilions, intensive care, and psychiatric units. I established a schedule for myself, each day covering a different pavilion or section of the hospital so that, by the end of the week, all Jewish patients have received at least one visit from me, with some patients, as needed, receiving two or three visits per week. Special requests for visits in critical or crisis situations were immediately honored, as were the cases of terminal patients. Messages from patients to whom I left my office telephone number, as well as from staff and outsiders related to the patients, reached me on my voice mail and emergency calls came via my beeper. The night administrator of the hospital also had my home number and called me on Sundays or in the middle of the night by phone. On the Jewish Sabbath and holidays when, as an Orthodox Jew, I am constrained from picking up the phone, they sent out a man from Security who knocked at my door, woke me up, and relayed the emergency message to me. I then followed him to the troubled patient and brought him relief in the middle of the night.

The two floors of our maternity units were visited regularly a minimum of twice a week according to special needs. The four sections of Psychiatry could and were visited regularly only by me, as family could visit there only at specific hours, and general visitors were not given easy entry. Finally, I visited with some non-Jewish patients who shared rooms with Jewish patients and indicated a desire to speak to me. When a non-Jewish hospital chaplain was absent or when a non-Jewish clergyman from out-of-town asked me to visit a sick parishioner at a time when one of our chaplains had gone home, I naturally obliged and then called him back with a report on the condition of his member.

I often stayed beyond official working hours. If I may say so, chaplaincy is far more demanding than being a clergyman in a community. However, it has its own rewards if you are dedicated to it and know how to be a real help to these suffering people.

I have been called a dedicated practitioner of my profession. This book, with its case histories – a first in publications – has a plethora of real problems actually faced by patients today and, for that reason, the language follows a conversational style, as the ability to enter into a meaningful dialogue with the patient is crucial. In this profession, which sees so much suffering, the chaplain must have the ability to evoke confidence and trust if his ministry is to be effective. Letters received by the administration and the chaplain usually describe the extent of the chaplain's support and influence. They constitute a true testimony.

To sum up the role of the chaplain, let me state that he has to be a warm person, a very caring person, a compassionate person, a wise and understanding person, a resourceful, innovative, and efficient person and must have what King Solomon prayed for: a *Lev Shomeya* – a listening heart, or in modern parlance, empathy to perceive the deeper needs of the patient and inspire confidence and faith. Then the chaplain can help the patient in his struggle for recovery and truly accomplish his task.

Some Practical Suggestions to Chaplains

Every chaplain must keep in mind that he will encounter people in crisis. I have my way of approaching a patient, and I have told it to many chaplains who worried about the first impression they will make on a patient. I just say: "I am Rabbi Spirn, head chaplain, and I came to wish you well." This usually gets the patient into a positive mood and he responds with a friendly, "Oh! Thank you." That opens the line of communication. The Code of Jewish Law, *III Yore Deah*: 335, and more clearly the *Kitzur Shulchan Aruch*: 193:3, defines the role of the visitor in the following way: "The essence of the commandment of visiting the sick is to look into the needs of the patient, what he needs to be done for him, and then, pray for his or her welfare." I have always kept that formula in mind as I approached a patient and I strongly recommend it to all chaplains. Try to assess what the patient needs, what you can do for him, verbally or concretely. We have two ears and one mouth. That may teach us first to listen well and sympathetically to what the patient has to say and then respond to or act on it. Only after you have done that, offer a prayer for a speedy recovery. I repeat: first, let the patient vent his feelings, unburden himself, with the chaplain just offering encouragement, sympathy, and a listening ear and then offer a prayer or pray with the patient. It is important to remember that the chaplain, most of the time, has easy access to the patient. So, if need be, work on his nonmedical problem and return to him and show him you have taken care of his problem to his satisfaction. Act as a friend. He will never forget that you were there for him and gave him real help when he needed it most.

Something more: Establish eye contact at all times. Bring a chair close to him. Keep your hand on his. Let him feel that what he says is of great interest to you, that you concentrate on him and will give him good advice, emotional support, or practical help. Your behavior will indicate to him that you are not just a person who has come to say hello to him *pro forma*, or tell him "God bless you" and leave. Keep in mind: Sick as he may be, he observes you carefully and weighs in his mind two options: to open up to you or to just be polite. Never challenge, contradict or argue with a patient. The hospital is not the place for that. Remember, you are there to help, to be friendly, to strengthen the patient's will to recover. Above all, do not play the doctor and do not advise about medical matters. Leave that to the physician, and you may be sure that when the physician will need your non-medical input, he will not hesitate to enlist your help – that is, if he knows you are a capable chaplain. In this book, you will find examples not only of patients trusting the chaplain but also of psychiatrists who did not hesitate to call upon the chaplain's wisdom and ability to make the patient cooperate, obey hospital and medical regulations, or even eat or shower.

A chaplain has to be nonjudgmental. When the patient is religious, that will be an additional reason for him to relate to you. At Mount Sinai, such a patient will also praise you for the religious improvements you may have introduced to make religious patients feel at home and at ease. I was blessed to have introduced seventeen projects, among which are: a kosher kitchen, after a hiatus of 124 years; a Jewish chapel enabling all Jews, including the most observant, to attend our services; five Jewish Sabbath elevators; a Sukkah and other projects. Some of those projects have served as models to other chaplains in the country and you too may wish to introduce some like them. As for those patients who tell you they are atheists or not practicing, do not be offended or argumentative. The hospital is not the place for that either. Try to speak to them about their health or personal problems they may want to discuss with you. Many times, too, they may talk to you about religious or transcendental problems, so point out explanations they may have overlooked or recommend books for their future reading. As an example, during some talks with nonbelievers who had high academic credentials, I told them about my French background and my doctoral dissertation at Columbia University which have not affected my religious observance. The dissertation was on Jean-Jacques Rousseau who, amidst deism and atheism of the eighteenth century, also had a positive attitude toward religion. That personal angle usually impressed them, and we parted in a very friendly manner. With wisdom and sensitivity one can thus have an intimate chat with many nonbelievers and the least that can be accomplished is gaining or increasing their respect for the religious tradition and friendship toward the chaplain.

Rabbi Dr. Charles A. Spirn

Statement: We did not mention the names of the patients who wrote letters or are mentioned in the case histories in order to protect their privacy.

C.A.S.

2: A CHAPLAIN'S PROGRAM AND INNOVATIONS

I feel that, as head chaplain, I had four functions:

- Making regular weekly visits to all Jewish patients plus additional visits as needed.
- Counseling patients, their families, and staff.
- Organizing and conducting religious services on Saturdays and all Jewish holidays and participating in all-year weekday afternoon services.
- Promoting the well-being of our non-Jewish patients through friendly personal rapport and referral to our multifaith chaplaincy staff.

In addition to my regular basic functions as head chaplain, I initiated and introduced to our hospital the following seventeen innovations of great importance to Jewish patients and staff:

- Jewish chapel where all Jews, including the most observant, can and do pray, built thanks to a very generous donation by philanthropists Stephen and Judith Peck. In addition, a separate Interdenominational chapel was built with the generous donation of Harold Ames Hatch.
- Kosher kitchen and cafeteria, supervised by the Orthodox Union.
- Five Sabbath automatic elevators.
- Passover night Seder, which drew two hundred attendees.
- Hanukkah celebration, including concert, which also drew two hundred attendees.
- Electric portable Sabbath candelabra for Klingenstein Pavilion and Klingenstein Clinical Center plus, at my request, six hundred Sabbath lights built into the headwall near each bed in our Guggenheim Pavilion, and seventy-two in our remodeled pediatric units.
- Patients provided with Kiddush and Challahs for Sabbath and holidays.
- *Eruv Chatzeroth* to enable observant people to carry in hospital halls during Sabbath.
- Advocate for observant patients to be free from signatures when being admitted on Sabbath and holidays. No discharge on those days.
- Complete *Megillah* reading on eve of Purim and daytime.

- Sukkah – booth on hospital premises.
- Ethrog and Lulav offered to patients, physicians, staff, and visitors.
- Adult Jewish education for staff – offering evening (5:30 P.M.) courses throughout the academic year. Our School of Medicine grants elective credit for Jewish studies to its medical students who take our courses.
- Mezuzahs placed at various entrances to hospital and to Jewish chapel, chaplain's office, and kosher kitchen.
- Resource person for continuously growing Judaica section in our patients' library.
- Arranging authorized visits by supervised young students on special Sabbath afternoons and holiday time (very well received by patients).
- Pre-Rosh Hashanah distribution of a few hundred Jewish-English calendars to administration, medical school, physicians, staff, and patients, in order to be aware of upcoming Jewish holidays and not schedule functions on those days and also to facilitate personal observance.

Indeed, every Jewish patient and staff member can now feel at ease and at home in our hospital.

We are also glad to note that hospitals and chaplains throughout the country turned to us for instructions on how to set up some of the above projects.

3: RELIGIOUS PROBLEMS AND NEEDS

"Rabbi – An Unanticipated Gift"

Director of Mount Sinai Hospital
5th Avenue & 100th Street
New York, N.Y. 10029
February 21, 1980

Dear Sir,

During my hospital stay at Mount Sinai for a back injury (December 13 to January 12) I planned to write you a letter of appreciation for Rabbi Spirn.

I am a writer and an analyst. The first sight of a rabbi in my room made me wonder scoffingly. Why a rabbi? A social worker, yes. But who needs a rabbi?

Until I observed the rabbi's total involvement with patients in my room, his complete dedication to giving them his unique moral and spiritual support. When I told him I planned to write an article on Ezekiel, he lent me some books from his own library.

The Sabbath morning service, attended by us patients, each in a wheelchair, was for me one of the most meaningful experiences in my life. His sermon, couched in his scholarly, skillful manner, in exquisitely beautiful English, was delivered to us as if he were addressing an audience of a thousand. And when he wheeled each of us up to the Torah for an individual blessing, I was moved to tears. His very presence, and his sincere devotion, instilled hope in me.

Meeting such a Rabbi in a hospital was an unanticipated gift. I thought you'd like to learn about it from one very grateful patient.

Sincerely yours,

Speed or Direction?

Every patient wants to get well and go home. At times, however, we find impatient patients who feel disappointed at not being discharged on a specific day and tend to become depressed. My answer to those patients is the following: Imagine two cars running on a road. One goes at 50 miles an hour and the other at 30. Now, the one that goes at 30 will surely reach the goal of the other eventually – a little later but he will get there *if he travels in the same direction*.

The same holds true about your health: What is basic and what I am concerned about is that you travel in the right direction, toward improvement of your health. If you do so, I am pleased, even if it takes a few more days. For what really and truly counts is direction and not speed. So, stop lamenting. Be satisfied that you are going in the direction of recovery. Just buckle up and do your best.

This approach, in my experience, has had a calming effect on patients and restored their perspective.

"Chaplain's Chaplain"

Dear Rabbi Spirn:

Thank you ever so much for sharing with me your years of service to the Jewish patients and their families at Mount Sinai Hospital. Your annual report contains a mere glimpse of the great humanitarian work you have done. The administration and staff of your hospital can indeed be proud and feel blessed that they have a man like you to serve them.

I know first hand how helpful you have been to me when I have called on your advice. Seeing you at Bikur Cholim meetings and those of the national Jewish chaplains, we all know how invaluable your assistance is. You can be looked upon as a "chaplain's chaplain."

May He above bless you with many healthy years to be able to continue with your noble and much needed services. Thank you.

Very truly yours,
Rabbi ---
Jewish Chaplain

Panic at Operating Room Door

An urgent message reached me that a patient on the verge of being wheeled into the operating room had panicked and insisted on seeing me first. I reached her promptly in the holding area of Annenberg 7, right at the threshold of the operating room. She had seen me during my regular visits and now, worried and frightened by the forthcoming surgery, wanted me to pray for her. I offered to pray the *Shema* with her and some other comforting and reassuring prayers and then added my own prayer. It all had a calming effect on her. She asked if she could take the Hebrew-English card from which we had prayed into the operating room. I left her, confident in God's mercy and watchfulness over her during surgery. My last words to her were that I planned to see her the next morning in her room and expected her, with God's help, to keep our appointment.

Presurgery: "He is a nervous wreck."

He had checked in only one hour before, and the nurses had a hard time handling him. He clamored for a rabbi. I was told on the phone: "He is a nervous wreck. Please see him right away." As I visited him, he admitted to being very nervous. He had never been a patient in a hospital, and now, at an advanced age, he was due for surgery the next morning. We talked about his operation, which is considered minor. I explained to him that he would not feel a thing, and that when he awakened, he would be in the recovery room. Then, within a few days, he would be discharged and be able to run to his synagogue on the forthcoming Rosh Hashanah. He had been in the needle trades most of his life, so I suggested humorously that he'd better let the surgeon do the sewing this time. As he gradually relaxed, I offered a special prayer for his well-being and the success of his surgery. Wanting to display his Jewish background, he spelled out for me his first name in Hebrew. I left him with a prayer text and with a scheduled appointment for the next day, following surgery.

Indeed, this presurgery fear is common even among the bravest people, and the presence of a clergyman does bring a great measure of relief. In this case, I used some light-hearted humor as I held his hand in mine for he was very tense, and I had to ease that tension.

"I Have Been Waiting for a Rabbi to Come"

These were her first words as I entered her room. I sat on a chair close to her bed and listened to a litany of troubles. She and her two teenage daughters had been in a car accident. The daughters have mercifully recovered from paralysis. She, however, was still having a problem with one arm when, unexpectedly, cancer was discovered in her body. She so much wanted to live! I let her verbalize her feelings and assured her I would carry out her request that special prayers be offered for her and her daughters. She too wished to pray, she said, but did not know how. I gave her some prayer texts, offered comfort, and, in parting, told her that I was going to watch over her through frequent visits and telephone conversations. The reaction was immediate: "Please do watch over me. I need it so much."

Back to Center

She was anxious and in tears. One eye was bandaged due to surgery, and she was terrified over the prospect of losing her sight altogether. There did not seem to be any medical reason for this fear of total blindness. I let her voice her fears and listened patiently. Then I described to her the extreme position she had taken by fearing the worst possible situation and urged her to get back to center, adopt a more realistic attitude that, with God's help, she would retain her eyesight – at least in one eye. Our exchange brought her some peace of mind.

The Patient Who Did Not Want to Recover

This patient kept pulling out the life-supporting tubes from his body, and his wife solicited my help. The patient was a religious man. I kindly but firmly alerted him to the Torah's prohibition against self-injury. I got across to him that life was both a gift from God and an obligation. Slowly, he calmed down and promised me that he would not interfere anymore with the efforts of the physicians and the nurses to save his life. I left him with a blessing for his speedy recovery. A son-in-law of this patient, religious and wearing a skullcap, followed me into the hall and told me that his father-in-law very badly needed this type of talk by a rabbi and thanked me profusely for my intervention.

Afraid of a Pacemaker

This seventy-two-year-old patient was afraid of the pacemaker that was going to be placed into his chest in a few hours, and he asked for the rabbi. When I entered his room and introduced myself, he requested that I pray with him. We prayed together, then we talked. After a while, he promised me to stop crying and to try to be as relaxed as possible, letting God heal him through His co-workers, the physicians. I told him that after surgery, he would be in the Annenberg Building, and I promised that at about 4:00 P.M. I would come there to speak to him again. He felt reassured. He had not wanted his wife to be informed about his impending surgery, so I was the only person in whom he could confide on that momentous day. When I saw him later, we shook hands. He felt a sense of relief, and I left him the prayer book he had asked for in order to offer thanks to God.

Car Accident Survivor

This patient had been in a fatal car accident in which she herself had suffered no physical damage but had witnessed the instant death of her seventeen-year-old girl friend, the driver. The patient suffered from headaches and, being a paramedic, requested codeine. Her psychiatrist to whom I talked felt that her problem was psychological, since all the tests were negative, and he refused to give her codeine because it would lead her to request more and more potent types of pain killers. Whereupon, the patient told the physician, "The rabbi is a man of God. I will listen to him." I urged her to follow the physician's advice and promised to return the next day to see her again. I thus became her only support as her family was unable to visit her. The trauma of the shattering experience did not leave her. Yet, she made progress, and the chance to talk at length to a nonmedical person whom she trusted eased her anguish greatly and helped her come to terms with the terrible memory.

Not Religious?

After my initial introduction, the patient retorted: "I am not religious." My reply: "But you are Jewish, and so am I." Then, when I asked him how he was doing, he opened up and revealed a problem, which I helped him resolve. His final words: "You are the first person to really help me."

Vietnam Aftereffects

Following our Saturday morning services, a man in his twenties approached me. He told me he had been looking for a rabbi and requested a private conversation with me. He had fought in Vietnam and had received many medals for bravery. His problem: a buddy of his was captured by a group of Vietcong guerrillas who shot him on the spot while he himself ran away and saved his life. Since returning to this country, he felt guilty for having fled and, being on the verge of committing suicide, checked himself into the psychiatric ward of our hospital. He wanted badly to find out from a rabbi whether he was guilty for having fled and abandoned his buddy.

My reply was that he was outnumbered and unarmed and stood no chance of saving his buddy. All he would have accomplished would be to get himself killed too – so there would have been two casualties instead of one. Jewish ethics does not ask this of anyone. In fact, the Talmud deals with a similar problem. It speaks of two men in a desert with just enough water to enable one to survive till he reaches civilization. In such a case, the law is that the one who possessed the limited amount of water in his canteen should drink it alone and survive, and not that both should share it and both die (*"Chayekha Kodmim" – Bava Metziah 62a*). With this in mind, I told him, "It is very clear that you acted right in fleeing. You are completely innocent." The former G.I. felt relieved after the conversation, and I made him promise never to harm himself.

I did not stop at that point. I asked him if he was married and had children. His answer was that he had a wife and two small children, and he loved his family. Whereupon I asked him: "Do you think it right to make a widow of your wife and orphans of your children? Who will support, guide, and raise them? Now, do you see your total situation? You were a good soldier and did your duty to our country. Ethics and duty now require that you, whom God had let survive, take good care of yourself, help your loving wife, and raise your dear children. I pray that you get well soon and have a beautiful home life with those you love and who love you and need you."

He felt a great relief after our session and, after a relatively short time, was discharged.

Rabbi and Mensch*

It was recently my privilege to make the acquaintance of a rabbi who truly brings honor to his calling, and who is a real mensch besides. Beginning in early August I was hospitalized for almost two months in Mount Sinai Hospital for kidney disease, and there I met Rabbi Charles A. Spirn, head chaplain of the hospital. On my first Thursday there, he came up to my room and cheerfully asked, "Tell me three good things about Susan." I was taken aback by that question, but in fact it was a psychologically sound one, because it forced me to take the focus off my various complaints and concentrate instead on the better aspects of my life.

We immediately formed a warm relationship, and from then on he came each Thursday to talk with me and to bring me Anglo-Jewish newspapers and other material. We usually discussed Israel and found that our views coincided on the whole. The rabbi is Orthodox (I am not) but that in no way interfered with our friendly relations.

Each Sabbath morning he held a service in the community room, which I attended as often as possible. Some of the patients were at times highly emotional and tearful, and I admired the rabbi's ability to show warm sympathy, yet not to allow the service to be unduly disrupted. His sermons were always brief but informative.

He also gave me a small folder with a collection of prayers for various times of the day. These gave me much comfort during a difficult time. The rabbi is a superb psychologist: He always seemed to know just the right thing to say to me when we met, always finding something uplifting at bad moments.

Truly, Rabbi Spirn combines the best of his religious calling with a warmth and humanity that are greatly to be admired.

– Susan Faulkner

---

*Susan Faulkner, *Tenants' Voice*, (now defunct) Flushing, N.Y. December 1989.

Words of a U.S. Air Force Officer: "You Have Given Me Strength, Rabbi."

He requested to have a talk with me in my office and not in the room where his wife was a patient. Her physician had described her condition as grim. He wanted me to tell him how to get the strength to face his situation. His first wife had died of cancer, though the surgeon had promised recovery. As a result, he had given up his religious practice. And now, he was facing a tragic situation again with his second wife.

To his question of "Why?" I responded that we do not know. The greatest sufferer in the Bible was Job, and he also wanted an answer to the same question. When his friends tried to suggest possible failings of his, Job replied he did not commit any of those transgressions. He remained with his dilemma till God Himself asked him where he was when He created the world. In other words, human minds have limits and cannot know all of God's ways of ruling the world. The same holds true for all of us who certainly are less perfect than Job. What we do know is how to act. On that, the Bible is very specific. So I encouraged him to do the very best for his wife as long as God gives her life. I further told him to think of the happy events in his life, the wonderful children and grandchildren who were giving him great emotional support, and to open himself again to prayer, synagogue, and God. I further gave him material for spiritual solace, including prayer texts I usually distribute to our patients.

Then, he took out of his wallet a photo showing him in his uniform as a bomber in the Army Air Force during the Second World War. Whereupon I suggested to him the concept that now, in peace time too, he and I and others were all soldiers in God's army, doing God's will as described in the Bible, and trusting God's loving kindness.

"You have given me strength, Rabbi," he said in parting and walked out in a more self-assured step.

"Rabbi ... A Very Calming Influence"

March 31, 1996

Dear Rabbi Spirn,

My husband and I would like to thank you for your great help during my husband's recent stay at the hospital. Your concern and caring had a very calming influence on us, and made a very tense time much more tolerable. We wish you good health, and may you be able to continue your wonderful work for many years.

Best wishes for a joyful Passover to you and yours and with deep appreciation.

A Special Place in His Heart

February 1, 1996

Dear Rabbi Spirn,

A famous philosopher of the past once said that "Stars may be seen from the bottom of a deep well when they cannot be seen from the top of a mountain. So are many things learned in adversity of which the comfortable man dreams not."

The truth of this statement came upon me with full force when I was recently hospitalized at Mount Sinai and had the privilege of meeting you. Your stature in the rabbinic constellation grew higher and higher as I personally experienced the sincere warmth of your concern and your deep involvement with all matters that could bring comfort to the members of my family and myself.

From the deep well of the Cardiac Intensive Care Unit at Mount Sinai, I could see the clear picture of a genuine star from which shone the light of compassion and strength to those who needed it so desperately.

I shall remember my stay in Mount Sinai for many reasons: the excellence of its doctors and their staff, the efficient nurses and aides, etc., etc. I shall have a special place in my heart for its chaplain, a truly great and shining star.

Sincerely yours,
Rabbi ---

Prayer in Lieu of Medicine?

A nurse at our Cardiac Intensive Care Unit asked for advice on what to do when disciples of a Hassidic rabbi prevent her from offering him medication according to a schedule prescribed by the physician, on the excuse that the rabbi was praying now and that prayer was more important than medicine. I gave her two answers. One was to have me contacted and let me handle this situation. A second alternative was to give the rabbi a schedule in advance, clearly spelling out at what hours medication is to be given to him. The rabbi would surely arrange his praying schedule in a way that would not conflict with his medical treatment.

Helping a Dayan – a Religious Judge

This grand gentleman and scholar had been a patient at our hospital a number of times throughout the year. He requested that I help him put on his *tallith* (prayer shawl) and his tefillin (phylacteries) for prayer every weekday morning. Of course I obliged and received profuse thanks and blessings from the venerable dayan and his wife.

Man of Faith

This patient, a Holocaust survivor, spent weeks at our hospital and his wife nursed him constantly. He was a man of unshaken faith. Said he: "God does not [merely] help me. He does more than that. He does everything for me." Such pure faith, especially coming from a man who knows what suffering means, was really to be admired. And his devoted wife too shared fully in his faith. I came to offer comfort and left full of admiration for their profound and genuine confidence in God.

"Warm and Good"

> Sir:
>
> With regard to your wonderful head chaplain, Rabbi Dr. Charles A. Spirn, let me tell you something. To be a patient in the hospital, away from family on a holiday, is very depressing. But the program Rabbi Spirn produced for us patients was outstanding and made me feel warm and good.
>
> Thank you,
>
> ---

Symptoms of Normal Religious Practice

Toward the end of Passover, an observant patient was admitted to our psychiatric ward, and he indicated he would appreciate visitors. My son, Rabbi Nahum (Neil) Spirn, before visiting the patient, first spoke to the patient's psychiatrist. She mentioned that she was concerned because the patient had not showered or shaved and she felt this was symptomatic of his depression. My son informed her that the patient was merely observing Jewish law, which prohibits these activities on a holiday, and further, that she could well expect the patient to continue not shaving during the period of semi-mourning – Sephirah – which follows Passover. The doctor was pleased to know that these "symptoms" were not of medical concern. My son then assured the doctor that he would encourage the patient to shower at the conclusion of the holiday. The patient readily agreed.

Russian-Jewish Newcomer Eager to be Religious

She was a nurse in training who also was enrolled in college. She approached me as I made my rounds in Maternity where she worked and asked for prayers for lighting the Sabbath and Festival lights. After I gladly gave her a set, including explanatory notes and the prayers in Hebrew and their translation and transliteration, she requested a set for her sister and then for her mother. I admired her interest in religion since she had come from Russia only a few years ago. Afterward, she inquired about the possibility of making her husband undergo ritual circumcision and a religious marriage ceremony for the two of them. I referred her to the proper people.

Refuses Heart Surgery on a Religious Holiday

Though she did not look it, she was a very religious person. I found her in our Cardiac Care Unit, CCU, and provided her with a Haggadah booklet for the Seder nights, which she observed in her unit, as intensive care rooms do not allow their patients to leave the floor, even for the official Seder inside the hospital. She contacted me whenever she had a problem. One such problem came up when she was scheduled for heart surgery (valve repair) on the seventh day of Passover, Friday, April 5, which was a full holiday. She just refused to be operated on during a religious festival. I checked with her doctors, who consented to postpone the surgery till the following Monday but preferred not to delay as there is always a risk involved. I presented the situation to her, giving preference to Friday, but she would not hear of it. And so, she made the decision for Monday, regardless of the risk in postponement. Surgery did take place then, and I am glad to say that God mercifully protected her, and she is on the road to full recovery.

"Elopement" During Purim Services?

She was a young woman in Psychiatry who was Orthodox and wanted to attend our Purim services. Since her supervisor could not spare any nurse to accompany this "risk of elopement" (escape) patient, she wanted to deny her permission to attend the services. Therefore, I explained to the supervisor that such a denial would upset the young woman profoundly because she was taught since childhood that there is a religious obligation to attend Purim services. Moreover, the risk of elopement could be overcome in two ways: (1) I would ask a resident doctor to watch over the patient during our services, and (2) the patient herself knows that one must hear the *Megillah* reading from beginning to end to fulfill the religious requirement. That would be an internal restraint against leaving in the middle of the services. The supervisor accepted my explanation. I am glad to say that the young lady caused no problem and expressed pride in never missing Purim services. She also partook of our *hamantashen* after services and walked around with a smile on her face and self-contentment in her deportment.

Applying Jewish Law to Paralyzed Arm

This male patient had had a stroke. His family turned to me to put phylacteries (tefillin) on him every weekday morning. As we know, phylacteries are usually placed on the head and the left arm. Since the stroke affected the left arm, the question arose whether *halachically* (by Jewish law) a man is obligated to put tefillin on that arm.

If the arm is atrophied and no blood comes out, it is considered in Jewish law as "dried out" and as if one had the left arm "missing" and one would not put tefillin on the arm at all but make one blessing on the tefillin of the head only. However, if the arm was only paralyzed (the cause of which is not in the arm itself but in the brain, and the arm is alive and bleeds when pierced), he would don the tefillin as usual on the left arm too. (Reference: *Igros Moshe, Chaylek* 1, *Seman* 8.) The latter was the case with this patient, and I placed the tefillin on his arm and head, waited while he prayed, and then removed them every weekday. The patient was so glad to have been able to pursue his daily devotions properly, and so was his family that had turned to me for help.

Disposal of Severed Limb

A nurse called at the request of a patient to inquire as to how to dispose of an amputated leg according to Jewish law. My reply: The funeral director is to bury it in a grave reserved for the patient. No religious service is needed.

Last Rite Prayer?

This patient felt his time was up. He had a serious heart condition and was in our Cardiac CU. After I introduced myself, he asked me what kind of rabbi I was. When I told him I was Orthodox, he told me he was Conservative and asked that I close the curtain of his room and then said: "What do you call that final prayer, you know, the prayer one recites when life is threatened?"

"You mean the *Viduy*, the Confession?" I replied.

"Yes, that's it. Say it with me," he said with tears in his eyes. I felt I should not proceed immediately to reciting the Confession, for then he might think that I indeed considered him terminal. Instead, trying to reassure him, I told him I wanted to give him an English translation of what the Code of Jewish Law (III *Yore Deah* 338:1) says: "Many people confessed and did not die and some others who had not confessed did die. Reciting the Confession brings an extra merit in favor of the patient for it shows that he wants to be at peace with God." And I added: "God, in His compassion, has granted such people many additional years of life. My prayer for you is that God help you too recover." I put a skullcap on his head, and we then recited the Hebrew text of the Confession, following which I told him its meaning in English, translating the Hebrew word for "sins" by the English "shortcomings" so as not to upset him. I left him saying: "See you tomorrow." His health did improve, thank God. A week later, he was in a regular room, out of bed, alert and cheerful, remembering every detail of what I had said to him and being grateful for it.

"You handled me very well," he said while shaking hands. "Thanks a lot, Rabbi."

Cremation Problem

A nurse from an Intensive Care Unit paged me. The wife of a terminal patient requested to see me urgently. When I reached her, she told me of her plan to have her husband's body cremated, and she wanted to know my opinion on this subject.

In a low-key fashion, I gave her three reasons for not doing that. First, it is prohibited by the Jewish religion. Secondly, in the future, the family may wish to pray at his grave, and all they will have is a container of ashes. Thirdly, we all bemoan the tragedy of the Holocaust martyrs whose bodies were burned by the Nazis in crematoria. "And now, how can one plan to do the same to a loving husband? Think about it. I suggest you give your husband a respectful burial." After a while, her response was: "You have convinced me, Rabbi. I will do as you suggest."

Prayer Text in Russian

A beautiful prayer pamphlet, *Selected Prayers for Health and Recovery*, issued by the Chaplaincy Department of the New York Board of Rabbis in English, has now been translated into Russian. We have obtained a supply of copies, which we give out to the Russian-Jewish patients at our hospital. They are all surprised and most appreciative of this service done especially for them. Similarly, visiting cards, which we leave at the bedside of patients who are not in their rooms at the time of our visit, have also been translated into Russian. On these cards, I write my name and telephone number for easy reference.

Fully Appreciates Rabbi's Innovations

February 12, 1996

Dear Rabbi Spirn,

As a long-time member of the Committee on Religious Affairs of the Federation of Jewish Philanthropies, I had been aware of your untiring efforts, throughout the years, to create a kosher kitchen and install

Sabbath (and Jewish holidays) elevators in Mount Sinai Hospital.

But it is only recently that, as a patient in the hospital, I came to truly understand and appreciate the value of your achievements. The freshly cooked, reliably kosher food I received during my stay definitely contributed to my recovery. And the knowledge that my dear family which so lovingly stayed with me could also obtain kosher food in the hospital in the "Kosher Corner" or in kosher guest-trays on the Sabbath, greatly contributed to my peace of mind. And let me not forget the comfort I derived knowing that there were Sabbath elevators and my dear ones did not have to climb nine flights to visit me on the Sabbath.

All these are your achievements, obtained, I remember, through years of negotiations and struggle. I thank you, in my name and in that of all other observant patients, for having so significantly contributed to our comfort and recovery.

In addition, I personally want to thank you for your interest in my welfare and the solace your visits gave me. They were indeed priceless.

With gratitude and warm regards,

No Room in Hell

"Will I go to hell?"

"No. There is no room for you there."

This exchange takes place frequently and always ends with a smile on the face of the patient, especially those who need constant reassurance. A certain young woman, of Orthodox background and education, entered our psychiatric ward. Her psychiatrist shared the diagnosis of her illness with me and asked for my intervention. I spent weekly sessions with her, and we had many Saturday conversations at the conclusion of our religious services, which she attended. She felt confident with me.

I often used humor to ease her tension, to make her smile and to overcome paranoid manifestations. For instance, she feared that someone would kill her. How does one react to that? My response was to tell her humorously: "Well, there are seven million people in this city. Why would anyone bother to pick on you?" She smiled at that. At another time, this Orthodox patient, who was extensively educated in Judaism, expressed fear that she may not be really religious. I calmly reassured her that her doubts came from her worries about her illness and not from weakening of religion. "You are a fully religious young woman, and you surely know in your heart that you love to pray and to relate to God." Pointing to a Hebrew prayer book on her desk, I asked whether she had already prayed that day. She had not. So I encouraged her to pray and reminded her to include the extra prayer (*Oveenu Malkeynu*) as that day was a fast day (Tenth of Tevet). When I told her that I was fasting as prescribed by Jewish law, I gained esteem in her eyes. As time went on, she admitted that there was something bothering her, something that she could not identify. "That," I said, "is a good sign. It is a sign of health to realize that one has a problem. Your psychiatrist will help you to identify the problem and to overcome it." And so, week after week, I listened to her questions and worries and endeavored to steer her on the road to health and sanity.

Handling a Recalcitrant Patient

The nurse beeped me to come over urgently to handle a problem with an Orthodox patient at the Cardiac Progressive Care Unit in 6C. It turned out that he had refused to eat his breakfast and take his pills. The nurse was kind and compassionate and looked for a way in which to help the patient. As I introduced myself, he kept on talking successively in three languages: Hebrew, Yiddish and Russian. The gist of it was that he wanted neither food nor medication. I must add that he was at least partially confused. Realizing that soft talk would not do, I told him that if he persisted in his refusal to eat and take medication, he would aggravate his condition and may possibly undermine his life and health. Then, quoting Jewish law, I told him that would cause him to lose his share in the World-to-Come. ("*Hamabed atzmo lodaath.*") This admonition suddenly rendered him alert to what I was saying. I continued on a positive note by quoting to him the Talmudic statement that the Torah gave permission to physicians to heal patients and that he should abide by that principle. I then asked the nurse to give him his three pills in my presence. As I encouraged him, he swallowed his medication. I also called up his wife and asked that a family member come to help supervise him. The next day, as I returned to visit him, the nurse was happy and grateful. To the patient I added that if God intended him to be an angel and not eat, He would have given him wings. Since he had no wings, he'd better eat, get well, and go home. This time, both he and his wife smiled.

"Full or Abridged Version of *Megillah?*"

On my voice mail, there was the following question before Purim: "Do you read the full or abridged version of the *Megillah*? Please return my call." My answer to that caller was that I read the full text of the *Megillah* as required by Jewish religious law. The reason for that is that only the full text reveals the Divine intervention within the unfolding order of events. For that, the congregation must hear every single word of the sacred scroll. Moreover, many of our Jewish patients are knowledgeable in Judaism and ask for the correct fulfillment of the religious requirement. Of course, that patient attended our services, as did scores of others, and felt relaxed and contented. My talk before the reading and chanting of the *Megillah*, explaining its contents in modern terms as taught by Rabbi Joseph B. Soloveitchik, professor of Talmud and Jewish philosophy at Yeshiva University, was most appreciated by all who attended as all understood me. Indeed, we pride ourselves in amalgamating people of various backgrounds into a united congregation. Everyone felt good and uplifted by experiencing Purim with us.

Resolving Conflicts in Psychiatry

A Hassidic man was placed in the Quiet Room in Psychiatry where, so the nurses told me, one is allowed to wear only his pajamas and have no hard-covered books for fear of violence. Indeed, that patient had already thrown books at the nurses. I was called in to calm the patient and to find a solution acceptable to the hospital staff's rules and to him. A special nurse sat at the entrance to his room for observation.

I established a friendly rapport with the man and learned that not only was he very pious, which I well expected, but also that he had traveled to Eastern Europe to set up new tombstones on the graves of Hassidic masters because the former stones had been broken by vandals. We talked a great deal about his experiences and then I slowly brought the conversation to his conflict with the staff. It soon became clear to him that I was in sympathy with his practice of religion and would plead for him within the parameters of religion and the rules in the Psychiatry Department.

I assured him that his prayer shawl (*tallith*), phylacteries (*tefillin*) and hard-covered prayer book would be returned to him at the proper times for daily worship. In the meantime, I had both a soft-covered prayer book and a soft-covered Book of Psalms returned to him. His four-cornered small tallith (*tzitzis*) was more difficult to obtain. The nurses insisted on his not wearing anything but a skullcap and pajamas. So I reminded him of the Jewish religious law that states that the small tallith need not be worn at night and also that, in the absence of a four-cornered garment, one need not wear the fringes (tzitzis) (*Chovas Cheftza* and not *Chovas Gavra*). Gently, he handed over the small tallith to the nurses.

We chatted some more, and I recommended that he not create incidents since his religious needs would be respected. He listened carefully and obliged. I am glad to state that a few days later he was back in a regular room. And a short time afterward, he was "honorably discharged" and went home to enjoy the Passover holiday with his family.

Helped to Undergo Circumcision

Four Russian Jews who were part of our hospital's doctoral program have been helped to undergo ritual circumcision. In the former Soviet Union, this basic Biblical requirement for all male Jews was prohibited by a government that repressed religion. All of the four insisted on being identified as Jews. One also added that he rejected his father's secularism and atheism and wanted to be a fully practicing Jew. I referred all of them to an organization called Friends of the Refugees of Eastern Europe (FREE) that had their circumcisions performed by a qualified mohel in a Brooklyn hospital under the supervision of medical staff – all at no charge.

Atheist Reconsiders

This involves a young patient in his late twenties whose name on the plate was followed by the title "Ph.D." When I introduced myself as a rabbi and a chaplain, he retorted that he was an atheist. Undeterred by this unexpected response, I told him that he was a Jewish atheist, and since I was a Jewish rabbi, we had something in common: our Jewishness. However, since he did not seem to want to talk, I said that I came to wish him well and hoped for another occasion to relate to him.

The following week he was in a different pavilion. When, without recognizing him, I approached his bed, lo and behold, it was he who reminded me that he was the man who had said that he was an atheist, and he apologized to me for it. I told him that I had not been shocked, that I also had a Ph.D., and that my thesis dealt with the eighteenth century French Enlightenment, which prepared me well to deal with atheism – so that there was no need to apologize.

In our conversation, I recommended that he read Hertz's Bible and Commentary to learn the Jewish view on creation and evolution, which he thought were irreconcilable. We then talked about his illness. When, before leaving, I said to him, "May God heal you soon" and stretched out my hand to him, he shook it warmly.

Addressing Ordination Class

January 10, 1995

Dear Rabbi Spirn:

Many, many thanks for presenting the chaplaincy in such meaningful fashion to our first year semika (Ordination) students.

I ask the students on their final exam to write a few sentences about the chaplaincy and whether they would see themselves in a hospital setting.

Many of them write very positively about your lecture and materials as having helped them in their understanding of the program and their positive attitude toward consideration of the hospital chaplaincy as a career. I know you will be as pleased as I with their response.

My best wishes to you and your beautiful family.

Sincerely,
Dr. Israel Miller
Senior Vice President
Yeshiva University

From Deism to Judaism

I found his name on the list of patients without a religious identity and felt that he could be Jewish. Indeed, when I visited him, he told me that his parents were Jewish but that he considers himself to be a deist and has his own relationship with God, requiring no synagogue. The family's rabbi, he added, considers him an atheist.

I soon noticed that he was a bright young man. He told me he was a prelaw college student. Responding to his interest in religion and his questions, I analyzed for him the concepts of deism, theism, and monotheism – areas with which I am especially familiar from my studies of the eighteenth century French Enlightenment. He asked pertinent questions and was honest and sufficiently objective to grant me that I made a point whenever he thought so. He was very attentive to my presentation of additional concepts, such as Jewish identity, organized and private prayer (he had believed only in the latter), the Sabbath and the code of kashruth. He had raised all these issues, to which I responded in a kind of Socratic dialogue, at the end of which he discovered himself to be completely in the orbit of Judaism.

We had spent an hour in the mutual intellectual stimulation during which he made the discovery of Judaism and the self-discovery that he believed in so many of its fundamentals. At his request, I left him with a list of books for future readings and study and, need I add, a sense of growth into new horizons.

Guest in Rabbi's Home

Dear Director:

Just recently my wife had need of hospitalization and was confined at Mount Sinai. During this difficult period, we both had the pleasure of meeting Rabbi Spirn, the chaplain on your staff.

My wife had surgery on Friday, April 14, and as we are both observant in our faith and dietary laws, we wanted to be as close as possible on the Sabbath. When Rabbi Spirn heard of my plight, he immediately invited me to his home for Friday and Saturday meals and provided me with a room on Friday night, so that I not only did not have to travel on the Sabbath, which the Jewish religion prohibits, but was close at hand to my wife all day Saturday – the time so important to her recovery. Apart from the spiritual comfort gained from meeting with the rabbi, his and his wife's generosity and kindness were a treasure.

My wife has since recovered from her surgery, and I wish to express my gratitude and hers for the professional manner and tender care your staff afforded her. As we both know, hospitals are not a place to be; however, when you must be confined, it is truly a delight to be treated so well by people you only just met.

My compliments to you as director and many thanks to your wonderful caring staff.

Most sincerely,

Early Morning Call

At 2:30 A.M. my home phone rang. In the Coronary Care Unit a patient was very depressed and cried ceaselessly. My intervention was solicited. When I entered that patient's room, I greeted him warmly and reminded him of my visit to him the day before.

"I am dead," he moaned.

"Well, the dead cannot speak – so you are not dead," I replied.

Slowly his presence of mind returned, and he apologized for his crying in the middle of the night. "The fact that you remember what happened is a good sign," I encouraged him. He had had heart surgery before and that worried him. I gave him reassurance that the staff felt his condition was stable, and it did not look as if he would need surgery again.

As he kept on expressing fears which were not justified, I asked him, since he was a very religious man, where was his trust in God. He then shifted to complain that the hospital had no Jewish chapel. "That's coming. It will take another year for our newest building to be completed," I answered him. "In the meantime, please remember the words of Psalm 115: 'You who revere the Lord, put your trust in the Lord! He is your help and your shield.'" Those verses calmed him down. I then offered the formal Hebrew prayer for the sick ("*Me Shebayrach*"), personalizing it by inserting his name into it. He listened carefully and then, reminding him that God was his helper and protector and, therefore, he should relax and trust, I shook hands with him and left. Said his grateful nurse to me, "It took a rabbi to calm him down."

Young Woman in a Prolonged Coma

This young Russian-Jewish woman, a specialist in the restoration of works of art, had gone into a coma and had stayed some four months at our hospital. Her widowed mother stood at her bedside every day of the week. We prayed for recovery and also offered solace to the mother, who spoke Yiddish but no English. I was able to get her some financial help, which she needed badly since the daughter had been the breadwinner for both of them. I also interceded in her behalf with JASA of Astoria about her rent. Above all, she needed someone to give her emotional support. I kept up my contact with her even after her daughter was transferred to Goldwater Hospital on Roosevelt Island.

It gladdens me to report that suddenly the young woman awoke. She speaks and eats and even plays Mozart again. We hope and pray that the damage to her brain is minimal.

Teaching Hebrew Reading

She was a fifteen-year-old patient at our hospital and after attending our Sabbath service, she expressed regret at not being able to read the prayers in Hebrew. I offered to teach her Hebrew reading so as to enable her to follow the Hebrew part of the service. Luckily, our patients' library had a beginner's Hebrew textbook and so, in the hall of her floor, we sat and studied. She grasped the material very quickly, and at her discharge was able to read Hebrew well. She was so proud of her accomplishment that, in telephone conversations with her parents, she demonstrated to them the Hebrew vocabulary she had acquired in our sessions.

"Services Made Me Very Proud to be Jewish"

> We had our Jewish Holy Days services on Rosh Hashanah and Yom Kippur and enjoyed them very much. The services, conducted by Rabbi Spirn, were beautiful. They made me proud to be Jewish. Thank you for making my stay at the hospital during the High Holy Days so very pleasant.
>
> Sincerely,
>
> ---

Lady Wants a Torah Thought

Her nurse left a message on my voice mail saying that this patient wanted to see me and would also appreciate a religious message. I responded to that call and, after talking for a while about her illness, she asked me for a *dvar Torah* – some instruction or elaboration on a Biblical text. Of course, I was glad to oblige and soon discovered that she had organized an adult education class in her home, taught by a rabbi. She herself was well educated in Judaism and her eyes livened up whenever I taught her an original Torah thought. Thereafter, every time I saw her, a *dvar Torah* became part of my visit.

Not to Tell

Looking at him, one would never guess that, according to his physician, he was only given three months to live. His appearance was that of a healthy man and his spirits were excellent. In the hall, his daughter revealed to me that her father had cancer and that the physician felt he should tell him the prognosis. The patient's wife and daughter, however, were fiercely opposed to his being told the brutal truth for fear it might well cause a complete deterioration of his condition and hasten his demise. They wanted to know my advice. I told them that in the Bible, the term "truth" (*emeth*) is always preceded by the term "lovingkindess" (*chesed*) to teach us to be careful when we are inclined to tell a destructive truth, which will accomplish nothing positive. My advice is not to tell the patient but make him spend the time allotted to him by God in as comfortable a manner and as loving an environment as possible. Do your best for Dad and leave the rest to God. The daughter, after having received rabbinic advice, felt surer of herself and more at peace with her position.

Love for a Grandfather

Her grandfather had been a patient at our hospital for a few weeks. Though she lived in Ohio, this young married woman came to New York for a few days to offer love and attention to her sick grandfather. For the Sabbath, we offered her hospitality in our home, so that she was able to visit with her grandfather on a holy day as well. Upon returning to Ohio, she sent us a card in verse, which she had composed for us. It read:

Dear Rabbi and Mrs. Spirn and Nahum:
Thank you for
sharing your home,
Making me feel
as one of your own.
You gave of yourselves
beyond all measure.
This to me is
the greatest treasure.
May abundant blessings be yours.

"Will You Pray for Me?"

Many patients make this request verbally. In some instances, patients who have undergone throat surgery and cannot talk write out the same request on their pads. I then ask for the patient's and his/her mother's Hebrew or Yiddish names and promise to oblige. The patient gains a sense of relief. Someone who cares will intercede before God in his/her favor.

"I Feel Good in Your Presence"

Following our Saturday morning service, this psychiatric patient who was knowledgeable in Judaism asked if I would return later for she felt good in my presence. I thanked her for the compliment and promised to see her during the week.

Surgery Not Needed Anymore!

She called me for an urgent visit. When I arrived, she began by telling me that she was not a religious person but that something extraordinary had happened to her, and she must share it with me, a rabbi. She had a blockage in an artery behind her knee and dilation attempts proved unsuccessful. Bypass surgery was then recommended. She was taken to the operating room and was administered anesthesia. Then, suddenly, she was awakened and told that surgery was no longer necessary. The anesthesia apparently moved or dissolved the clot in the blocked artery and circulation started again normally. This nominally nonreligious patient called it a miracle. It certainly was something to marvel about and be grateful for. At her request, I offered a prayer of thanksgiving. Having been spared surgery and its aftermath, she felt grateful to God and decided to light Sabbath candles and also offer her own thanksgiving prayer every week.

A Treat in Psalms

This lady, a vivacious patient with a cheerful spirit, insisted on reciting to me numerous Psalms in English, which she had memorized through the years. In perfect diction, it was just a flow of texts, one after the other. She considered herself religious in her own way and had developed a love for the Psalms in which she was so fluent. As she declaimed them in English, I followed her with the Hebrew text in my mind. She had a good translation. I learned from that case that one also comforts a patient by giving the patient one's attention and letting the patient express herself and display her knowledge. She just beamed, and I felt glad for her.

Praying in the Clothes Closet

This very pious rabbi, a patient in our hospital, felt it was not respectful to pray to God in a room having urinals. He, therefore, prayed in his prayer shawl (tallith) and phylacteries (tefillin) in...his clothes closet! I cautioned him about the danger of locking himself accidentally in that closet, yet he persisted. What he wanted was permission to pray in a clean room on the floor. I obtained permission for him to use the treatment room and thanked our nurses for their understanding and cooperation.

Hemodialysis Unit

I regularly visit the Jewish patients in our Renal Department and, when necessary, I see them during dialysis as well, when a friendly face and a kind word are highly appreciated during those long sessions.

Anxiety over Not Kissing the Mezuzah

She identified herself as not too religious a person. She declined my offer to provide her with an electric candelabrum to kindle the lights for the Sabbath. Yet, she expressed her worry and fear for having forgotten to kiss the mezuzah when she left her home to go to the hospital.

The mezuzah is a tube appended on the doorpost of the home, and it contains passages from the Scriptures. When one enters or leaves the house, one touches the mezuzah and then kisses the fingers. The mezuzah is a religious symbol signifying that God is welcome in that house.

This patient was due for surgery the next day and became apprehensive because she forgot to touch the mezuzah, which meant that she did not invoke Divine blessings on her trip to the hospital. The solution I offered her was to recite the *Shema* prayer ("Hear, O Israel") which is the beginning of the text inscribed on the parchment in the mezuzah. I gave her a card containing the prayer and thereby enabled her to regain her confidence and trust.

"Please, God, Give Me a Second Chance"

He was a patient for long weeks and requested that I visit him often and pray for him. He badly wanted to recover, and yet felt guilty about his past life. He had a fairly good Jewish background but was not religious at all. Realizing his medical condition, he pleaded with God for just another chance. He promised to act like a new person and in consonance with Jewish tradition. I offered him comfort, repeated to him that teshuvah (repentance) helps, and encouraged him in his new resolutions. He was discharged from the hospital and has not returned. Hopefully, he is doing better, medically and otherwise.

Request: Judaic Studies Tutor

A social worker called about an unusual problem: a chronically ill twelve-year-old boy in our Pediatric Pavilion wanted a Hassidic tutor to give him lessons in Judaic studies at our hospital. Luckily, such a tutorial service does exist, and I was aware of it. The Chai Lifeline of Brooklyn does provide a free tutor at hospitals for Jewish students, ages five to eighteen inclusive. The tutor prepares the child for his return to the classroom and later helps him to catch up with his classmates. I was very glad to be able to refer one young patient to this service organization.

"You Are Still Needed"

He said he had a question for me. He was in pain and in a bad state of mind. Why did he survive the Holocaust when thirty-two members of his family perished? he asked.

"You are needed in this world. You still have a job to do," I responded.

"What job?" he inquired. To that question, I replied that he has to look into his own life and find out what good he could still do. At this point, he became reflective. I had directed his mind to search what he could do for God and for people. He also became more relaxed.

Hypocrisy? No!

As a service to our patients, we offer electric candelabra for igniting lights for the Sabbath. Occasionally, a patient responds that she had never lit the Sabbath candles and does not want to be a hypocrite by lighting them now. My reply usually is that the characteristic of a hypocrite is to be a deceiver. "In your case," I tell the lady, "you certainly have no intention of deceiving anyone. You are not deceiving God, you are not deceiving yourself, and you are not deceiving me. I recommend that you read a play by Molière called *Tartuffe*. There you will see a real hypocrite, a real deceiver. But you are not that. A good deed comes your way, and you just do it. It is a religious act – true. Aren't we all praying for God's blessing and healing?" The response I get is positive. Truly, we are all what Jewish tradition calls us – believers and descendants of believers.

Correct Date of His Mother's Yahrzeit

He said he had a question for me. His mother died six years ago and he was observing her Yahrzeit (anniversary of death) every year on a different date since he did not know the Hebrew date of her passing. He felt troubled by that. I promised him prompt help. I looked up the Hebrew date of her death in an English-Hebrew calendar, which will enable him to observe the correct date this year, and every year in the future. This brought him great relief.

Faculty Meeting Shifted

An important meeting of Medical School faculty and senior administrative staff had inadvertently been scheduled by the dean's office for the afternoon of the second day of Rosh Hashanah. This led many physicians and other invited staff members to visit me, to leave voice mail messages, and to write to me – all asking for my intervention. I am glad to state that the office of the dean also called and checked dates with me. As a result, the inadvertent mistake was rectified and the meeting was rescheduled for the next morning after the holiday. I wish to express our thanks to the dean for being sensitive to Jewish susceptibilities and practices. I have also presented him with a new Hebrew-English calendar to help with future scheduling.

"I Was in Heaven"

With a serious mien, this patient declared to me, "I was in heaven." Asked for an explanation, he related that his heart had stopped beating. Luckily, he had recovered so well that he was ready to return home seven days after heart surgery. Remarkable indeed! Usually patients are not ready to go home until ten days have passed. His room had flower vases and his walls were filled with get-well cards. I left him with the comforting thought that obviously he was loved by people and loved by God.

"Services by Rabbi Contributed to My Health and Sense of Well-Being"

August 22, 1994

Dear Director:

I have the all too frequent opportunity to spend a few days at Mt. Sinai due to my treatments for cancer. Many people at all levels of your organization have helped to make my experiences more comfortable, secure and optimistic. When I seek spiritual support, I am more concerned with the expertise and capability of those who are helping me rather than asking for a miracle to change my condition.

The efforts made on my behalf by those employed and in voluntary service at Mt. Sinai show me that my prayers are answered in small, great, heroic and unnoticeable ways.

I have had the opportunity to visit the synagogue located at Mt. Sinai on two occasions and although I am, at best, a casually religious person, I have found these visits to hold great meaning and fortification for me. The services conducted by Rabbi Charles Spirn have contributed to my overall health and sense of well-being. I am thankful to the hospital and the directors for providing this opportunity to approach our faith during these especially difficult times of need....

Best regards,

---

cc: Rabbi Dr. Charles Spirn

Elective Credit Granted

An exceptional innovation I have introduced at our hospital was the creation of Adult Jewish Education classes, which took place on Mondays through Thursdays from 5:30 P.M. to 7:00 P.M. on our premises. Classes included: crash courses in reading Hebrew with emphasis on prayer book Hebrew; modern conversational Hebrew on three levels; crash courses in basic Judaism; Bible: the Pentateuch; post-Biblical Jewish history; modern Jewish history; Jewish mysticism and Kabbala; the Bible and us: a taste of Torah; a taste of Kabbala; study of book of mysticism: *The Way of God* by Moshe Chayim Luzzatto.

I ran those courses for eight years, partly in conjunction with the National Jewish Outreach Program of New York. Interestingly, our School of Medicine granted elective credit to its medical students who took our courses. They had to use tailor-made forms from the Office of Student Affairs, which were signed by the instructor.

Unusual Requests by Staff

- She was Chinese-American, an employee of our hospital, and her daughter followed an American program at the Tel Aviv Medical School. Since the daughter will be spending her vacation here, she would like to be tutored in Hebrew. I located a teacher of Hebrew to give her private lessons.
- She was of Russian-Jewish background and was employed at our hospital. She was deeply concerned about her nineteen-year-old nephew in Moscow, who became religious and struggled on his own to find kosher food, which, in addition, was especially expensive. Her request to me was to find someone who goes to Russia and could be of some help to that young man. After some research, I found an organization called Coalition for Soviet Jewry that is in touch with the Moscow Synagogue and with its American rabbi who is the Chief Rabbi of Moscow and helps people like that young man.

Letter From a Friend

October 25, 1990

Dear Rabbi Spirn,

This letter is long overdue but I was busy "taking good care of myself" (as you advised me to do) and now that I feel a lot better, it is time to tell you how much you contributed to my well-being at Mount Sinai Hospital, professionally and more so as a friend.

The meals were, of course, very appreciated, especially on Shabbos and Yom Tov. I have told you repeatedly how nicely prepared they were. But I can't begin to tell how much your visits, your care and concern meant to me. They did my mending heart much good.

In friendship,

An Unusual Hassidic Custom

A custom practiced by many Hassidic Jews following the week of mourning (*shivah*) over a deceased member of the family is to return to the deceased's hospital room or just stay at its door, recite Psalms and pledge charity. They do so as an act of bringing peace to the soul. If the room happens to be unoccupied, there is no problem. However, if occupied, the Hassidim are very careful not to upset the present patient. They just stay in the hall near the door, and all one notices is that they are holding a prayer book in their hands and praying silently. If, however, they learn that the present patient is in fair health and in good spirits, they just wish the patient well and ask permission to use the sink for washing their hands and, in the process, offer a silent prayer and pledge of charity. This is a very delicate matter, and I witnessed it once only when they talked to a nurse about it. That time, I assisted them in handling it unobtrusively and with utmost care.

"You Brought Me Relief"

Her father, an elderly patient at our hospital, was terminal. He was a religious person and the family wanted to make sure no one except the members of the Holy Society (*Chevrah Kadisha*) should touch him after his death. She had sleepless nights, she said, worrying about this problem, and decided to ask for the hospital chaplain. Instead of talking over the phone, I decided to go to her father's room and let her express her worry personally. I then offered a solution and had it immediately implemented: I had a nurse insert a note into the patient's chart expressing the family's wish. "You brought me relief. Thank you," was her reply.

Electric Thermometer on the Sabbath

I was called over to the nursing station of our maternity ward on a Friday to resolve a problem. The husband – a rabbi and teacher at the advanced Lakewood Yeshiva – pleaded with the supervisor not to use an electric thermometer on his wife during the Jewish Sabbath. My solution that he buy a plain oral thermometer for his wife and that the nurse use it when she has to take the patient's temperature was readily accepted. Religion and medicine were happily reconciled.

Another Chance with Grandchildren

A number was tattooed on his arm – a sign that he had been in a concentration camp. He had surgery and was recovering nicely. But he needed someone to talk to in order to relieve himself of what was oppressing him. He was a religious man and had given his daughter, whom he described as highly intelligent, a complete general and Jewish education. Now she was married to a professional whom he also described as highly intelligent. But now the shock: She did not keep a kosher home, so all he could take there was a cup of coffee. Tears came to his eyes. He had done everything possible to raise a religious child, and now he could not face the disappointment.

I let him unburden himself, and tried to console him by saying that return to religion is always a possibility. But what brought him a measure of comfort and hope was my advice to be close to and loving to his grandchildren and that what was lost by his daughter, his grandchildren might recover. This gave him a goal. He felt he had another chance. And so I left him with a blessing for success.

Comfort Following a Miscarriage

She was a young Orthodox woman in our maternity department and had just had a miscarriage. I offered words of hope and comfort. When there is a tree, I told her, there will be fruit. I also helped her to pray with special fervor the Sabbath prayer *Yekum Purkan* wherein we ask Heaven to grant us "offspring who will live." I left her with the quotation of that prayer, "*Zuroh Chayo Vekayamoh*," which she understood ("with offspring who will live"). I think I saw a smile on her face as I left. Indeed, she was very familiar with that Sabbath prayer, and it meant the world to her.

Help Improves Communication with the Physician

Her mother's physician had told her he would have to perform a tracheotomy but she had opposed it, and the physician had walked away. Now, she complained, she did not know what would happen to her mother. I advised, "Do not practice medicine without a license. If you really want to communicate with the physician, just tell him that you would appreciate his explaining to you how the tracheotomy would help your mom. Instead of arguing with the physician, just ask politely for information, and he will certainly give it to you." She did so and got to understand her mother's condition better.

Appreciation for Long Term Multiple Services

November 14, 1995

Dear Director:

First I must thank the Mount Sinai Medical Center for the excellent care provided to my father. My appreciation goes out to all involved with his care.

The prime purpose of this letter is about a very important person at Mount Sinai, a unique and great person: your esteemed rabbi, Dr. Charles Spirn, chief chaplain.

The space in this letter is not sufficient to describe every detail, since it will resemble an oversized chart.

Rabbi Spirn contributed to the comfort and ease my father needed for recovery, by visiting, talking, praying, providing weekly Jewish newspapers and magazines, providing Sabbath candelabra, kosher refrigerator, sleeping cot for myself and also served as Yiddish interpreter for the speech therapist. And countless major or minor requests, advice, counseling, etc. Rabbi Spirn was always there.

I observed Rabbi Spirn doing the same for other patients as well. Not waiting for them to ask him, but asking patients and their families if their needs were met. When in times of stress, emotion and pressure, some people were glad to be reminded and guided by Rabbi Spirn.

Most importantly, Rabbi Spirn has and is conducting pastoral services in Hebrew, English, and Yiddish so that patients and families from a broad spectrum of Jewish faith may join and participate.

I had the opportunity to pray in the Peck Jewish Chapel during the holidays of Passover, Shavuoth, Shemini Atzereth, and on Saturdays and was impressed by Rabbi Spirn's attention to every detail, such as giving religious honors to patients and that every man and woman is called upon to provide the name of a patient for prayer for the sick.

And a final elating note is the Sukkah Rabbi Spirn set up. Words cannot express the joy and admiration visible on all participants, Mount Sinai staff doctors, health care workers, students, patients, families, and visitors alike.

Mount Sinai has earned an excellent reputation as a world class health center. In the year 2002 it will celebrate the 150th anniversary of its founding, and Mount Sinai has contributed to other institutions guidance in chaplaincy only through Rabbi Charles Spirn. Thank you.

Respectfully,

Supporting a Distressed Family

I noticed that the family was particularly moved by the uncontrolled crying of a young lady who turned out to be a daughter-in-law of the patient. Problem: serious case of surgery. I spoke with the family and left my visiting card, which, in addition to my name and telephone number, also has verses from Scripture. Interestingly, a week later, when I visited that floor, the lady-patient was doing well and, from under her pillow, took out a Hebrew prayer book and my card and told me that both had been with her in the operating room. She thanked me for having brought relief and hope to her family and especially to her daughter-in-law, gave me her home address, and said, "I will do anything I can to help you in your important work."

Battered Wives

Occasionally I encounter battered wives who are patients on our psychiatric floors. I also receive calls from outside our hospital asking for guidance in such a matter. By a happy coincidence, there came to my attention a lecture entitled "Legal Remedies: Part of the Treatment for Battered Women." It was given to me for our hospital by the co-chairperson of the Governor's Task Force on Domestic Violence. I am glad I attended. Later, I forwarded the speaker's Handbook for Beaten Women and a reference reading list of thirty-four studies on this subject to a Jewish transition center for battered wives, which offers hospitality but was not aware of wider educational and legal aids available.

4: EFFECTS OF RELIGIOUS SERVICES

"Vision and Generosity"

October 8, 1990

Dear Director:

Because I have been with my sister at the Mount Sinai Hospital for several weeks, I have had the opportunity of attending the excellent Sabbath and High Holy Day services conducted by Rabbi Dr. Charles A. Spirn, your head chaplain. His services have been so warm and inspiring – and have been of great help to me in coping with my sister's illness. It seems to me that Rabbi Spirn has created an oasis of peace and religious healing in the midst of so much illness and suffering.

I feel sure that Rabbi Spirn is appreciated for his enormous contribution to the Mount Sinai Medical Center; Mount Sinai is to be congratulated for its vision and generosity in making Rabbi Spirn's fine services available to so many.

With many thanks, I am
Sincerely yours,

Rosh Hashanah and Yom Kippur

The High Holy Days' services are particularly special at Mount Sinai. They are held in our beautiful Peck Jewish Chapel. We drew a capacity attendance, spilling over to the hall, and still have a number of people standing in the aisles. First of all, our own patients join us, some in wheelchairs, plus members of their families. Joining us also are residents, medical students, nurses, and other staff. What is most special is the spirit that prevails during services. I am particularly moved by the fervent prayers of all the participants, and their complete attention to the explanations of those most moving prayers. It is a true religious experience, and throughout the services one can hear a pin drop, so perfect is the decorum. As one young woman said to me: "The services were most meaningful and relevant." And many letters reach us after the holidays thanking us for our inspiring services. Indeed, everyone is drawn into real praying, into spending those precious and sacred hours for deep introspection and raising one's soul toward Divinity.

As Viewed by a Worshipper

October 13, 1996

Dear Director:

Our adult son was a patient in the Guggenheim Pavilion from September 11 until September 16. We want to express appreciation through you for the excellent care he received during this interval. Aside from the quality of medical services, we are grateful for the pervading attention to the feelings of patients' families. The design, staffing, and other features of the second floor waiting room were particularly helpful during the period of our intense anxiety.

As observant Jews, we are especially thankful for Rabbi Spirn. He is unusually attentive to emotions as well as formal religious needs. We stayed close to our son at the hospital during Rosh Hashanah. It meant so much to participate in services at the chapel. During these services, we again admired Rabbi Spirn's solicitude for patients and their visitors as well as his erudition. He structured and led the services with great sensitivity for the needs of all who attended.

We feel proud to be part of the Jewish people whose genius for human and medical service is so well expressed at the Mount Sinai Medical Center.

Cordially,

Reply from the Director

November 4, 1996

Dear Mr. & Mrs. ---:

I read with great pride your letter of October 13, 1996. Thank you for taking the time to write such a warm and thoughtful letter sharing with me the details of your family's experiences at The Mount Sinai Hospital.

At Mount Sinai, we strive to maintain a standard of excellence in the provision of patient care with a strong emphasis placed on the needs of and sensitivity to the patients' family as well. Letters such as yours serve as a tremendous source of encouragement to management and staff alike in our efforts to achieve this goal.

I was particularly delighted to read of your high regard for Rabbi Spirn and your appreciation for him and the religious services offered at

Mount Sinai. By copy of this letter, I am sure he will be equally as pleased with your lovely sentiments. I have also taken the liberty of forwarding your letter to the operational and clinical directors for the General Medicine Care Center so that it too may be shared with the staff who cared for your son while he was a patient on 9 West.

Again, thank you for your letter. I wish you and your family good health and a speedy recovery.

Sincerely,

Director

CC: Rabbi Charles Spirn

Time off for Rosh Hashanah

A group of six Jewish dieticians turned to me for help in getting time off for Rosh Hashanah. I contacted the assistant director of Support Services, and we both agreed that an exchange of working days should be encouraged between dieticians whereby Jewish staff gets off on the Jewish High Holy Days and the Christian staff takes off on Christian holy days. The principle of reciprocity was voluntarily accepted to the satisfaction of all concerned.

I hasten to add that another solution is also available: our hospital gives staff four extra free days a year which many use for religious holidays. Our six dieticians had used up the four days for other purposes.

Urgent Call! Wants Maftir on Yom Kippur

Two days before Yom Kippur, a call came to me from the RCCU that a patient wanted to see me urgently. As I rushed to see him, I noticed he had a large Hebrew book with the Haftorahs of the year. He opened it on the pages of the Haftorah (passage from the prophet Isaiah, 57:14–58:14) that is chanted at the Yom Kippur services by one individual and asked that he be allowed to chant it. Since he was in a cardiac unit, I doubted whether he would be able to attend our chapel and, if yes, whether he should be exposed to the strain of chanting a fairly long text. Yet, on Yom Kippur, he did attend our services after he was moved from the Intensive Care Unit to a regular room. Moreover, he insisted on chanting the maftir, and a roommate of his mentioned that he had practiced a lot during the night. I let him have this honor, and he made his way slowly through the text of Isaiah. He was very proud of his accomplishment, and I am sure his feelings of satisfaction contributed to his physical improvement as well.

Yom Kippur with Us as Viewed by a Worshipper

October 4, 1996

Dear Sir:

I attended Yom Kippur services at your hospital, as my favorite uncle had just undergone extensive surgery and was still in the Intensive Care Unit. Thank you for providing these wonderful services to us, as I and my family wanted to be with my uncle and still have a chance to attend services.

Rabbi Spirn led a beautiful service. The rabbi's inclusion of historical references during the service were inspiring, thought-provoking, and educational, and his other comments were meaningful in content. Additionally, the length of the service was perfect: long enough to make one feel as a participant in the service, without being so long that one might feel neglectful of our precious patient.

The services were very well attended. Indeed, there was no room to spare. I was very touched by the number of patients in wheelchairs and hooked up to monitors and IV who attended. I can imagine how important and meaningful their attendance was to them, and I can only thank you again for providing them and the families of your patients with beautiful services in a lovely chapel.

Very truly yours,

CC: Rabbi Spirn

"Most Compelling Yom Kippur Service"

Dear Director:

You've got a tough job, but it's a lot easier when you have good people such as Rabbi Charles Spirn, Mount Sinai chaplain. We've known our doctor for at least twelve years. Dr. Spirn, of course, I did not know, but he made my stay last September over Yom Kippur particularly comfortable, as he performed the most compelling service we yet attended. Please accept the enclosed check earmarked for Dr. Spirn and his services.

Very truly yours,

Enclosure: $100

"A Deeper Appreciation of Judaism"

Dear Rabbi:

Thank you so much for your help! You are truly a gifted teacher and have helped me attain a deeper appreciation of Judaism. I am very grateful to you.

Best wishes,
---, Ph.D.

"Very Dignified and Instructive Services"

Dear Sir:

On Yom Kippur Eve and Day, I attended the services in the Mount Sinai chapel conducted by Rabbi Spirn.

I just want to express my appreciation for these services conducted in a very dignified and instructive manner.

My son was in the hospital and had major surgery the next day. He is recuperating nicely, and Rabbi Spirn's words were a real encouragement at that time.

Sincerely,

CC: Rabbi Spirn

Reactions of a Medical Student

October 8, 1992

Dear Director:

I want to thank you very much for the rabbinical services provided by Rabbi Dr. Charles Spirn at Mount Sinai. As a third-year medical student, it has meant a lot to me to be able to attend religious services here at Mount Sinai, but the convenient location has been only a small part of what has been so meaningful. Rabbi Spirn has been a very special person to me. He welcomed me to attend the religious services, invited me to attend the special classes that he has made available at the medical center, and has been kind and supportive throughout my medical school training.

The religious services are conducted beautifully. It is amazing that Rabbi Spirn is able to meet the needs of such an eclectic audience, ranging from the Orthodox to the very reformed. He explains everything in English, leads prayers in both Hebrew and English, reads from the Torah, delivers a sermon relating the Torah reading to contemporary life, and still finishes before the patients in attendance become too tired. All of this is accomplished within a remarkably short period of time, and amidst many distractions. Although there are far fewer distractions in the beautiful new chapel, he handles all potential problems in a very eloquent manner, without missing a beat. Rabbi Spirn shares a wealth of knowledge at these services. His discussions are provocative and apply to everyday life, which for me includes learning both the art and science of medicine. I feel very fortunate that I have had the opportunity to take advantage of this valuable educational experience.

Last fall, Rabbi Spirn encouraged me to take a Hebrew reading course, which was a lot of fun. The classes were taught by a Hebrew teacher, but Rabbi Spirn always stopped by to say hello, give us information about the upcoming holidays, and to obtain feedback about the course. I had planned on continuing with these courses last winter, but found myself completely overextended with my schoolwork. Rabbi Spirn was kind enough to call me at home to see if he could make any special arrangements for me to attend any of the classes. He even offered to tutor me on his own time. When he realized how overwhelmed I was with my schoolwork, he reassured me that my schoolwork was more important, for the time being, that he knew that I was a good student, that it was important for me to study hard, and that he was sure that I was a going to become a good doctor. I shall never forget his kindness in offering the tutorial, his support in encouraging me to study, his belief that I would pass my exams, and his reassurance that I would someday become a good doctor.

Rabbi Spirn has been not only a friendly face in the hallways of Mount Sinai, but also a valuable resource and role model for me. Rabbi Spirn represents a large part of what makes Mount Sinai so special to me.

Sincerely,

"It Is Good… to Know That You Are There"

September 2, 1993

Dear Rabbi Spirn:

Enclosed please find check for $250 toward the Jewish Chaplaincy Fund. I know you have been a great comfort to my friend and her family.

It is good for us who care to know that you are there.

Enclosed: $250

"I Have News for You"

Very often, we find patients who are sad and depressed at having to spend a holiday like Rosh Hashanah in the hospital, especially in one of our Intensive Care Units. It is clear that such patients will not be able to attend our religious services. After talking with them and with our staff, I usually offer an abbreviated prayer book or a regular mahzor saying: "I have news for you: There will be a Rosh Hashanah next year. So please pull yourself together and do your best for your recovery." Where permissible, the shofar will be blown in such units too. I find that this approach brings relief to patients who begin to feel that everything has not been lost. There is some practice in the present and hope for the future.

Religion and the Use of Catheters

I received an unusual request from our oncology and surgery departments. It involved the use of two types of catheters: one the Broviac or Hickman catheter which is hooked up to the skin (venous access), remaining outside the body, and the other, newly marketed, called the Port-a-Cath, which is implanted under the skin. The experience of our physicians has been that Hassidic patients, for religious reasons, insist on the latter type – and the doctors wanted to know what they were. I replied that Hassidic people – men and women – go regularly for purification in a mikvah (a special pool of natural water for ritual immersion and purification). During the immersion, there must be no adhesive matter on the body, for it may prevent the water from reaching every part of the body. While the Broviac catheter is on the surface of the body, causing a separation between the body and the water, the Port-a-Cath is completely under the skin and is, therefore, selected by the Hassidim. Moreover, going to a mikvah with a Broviac catheter runs the medical danger of contamination, as water would enter the catheter, so a Port-a-Cath is clearly the better choice in these cases.

Moving on the Sabbath?

She was a very observant woman, and she strenuously objected to being transported by elevator on the Sabbath to a higher floor. She asked for my intervention. The staff gave two reasons for immediate transfer: The bed on the other floor may be given to another patient and, after 4:00 P.M. on Saturday, the transportation staff is restricted. Nonetheless, I must say, to the nurses' credit, that they listened to me and the moving was done after the conclusion of the Sabbath.

"Visits Brighten Day" – "Passover Seder Extraordinary"

Dear Director:

My mother has been hospitalized at Mount Sinai twice in the last year, and I am writing to you at her request about Rabbi Dr. Charles A. Spirn, Mount Sinai's head chaplain.

My mother and I feel a great deal of gratitude toward Rabbi Spirn for all his attention, which has made her cope so much better with her illness. He has arranged for her to go to Sabbath services, whenever possible, and to get regular visitors and kosher "noshes" from outside organizations. He also brings her electric Sabbath candelabra and Jewish-subject newspapers. His visits always brighten her day, and all his kind gestures are much appreciated.

It's especially important, I think, to compliment Rabbi Spirn on the extraordinary Passover Seder, which he led so capably. I had the pleasure of attending with my mother, her "roommate," and an aide. It seemed an enormous undertaking, but was well organized: I could see plainly that virtually everyone in that great crowd participated and enjoyed themselves – some even came away more enlightened.

I enjoyed his wonderful explanations of the holiday, its history, and how it relates to the contemporary world and current events, which helps make apparent what Judaism is: a very beautiful, modern, and timeless religion.

The now-famous Seder is a particularly important religious and social event for patients and their families; I sincerely hope that it will continue for as long as the rabbi is willing to do it.

With our heartfelt thanks to you for providing the hospital's patients with these and other such valuable people and benefits – in addition to the necessary medical ones to more surely help patients toward recovery.

Very truly yours,

"Makes Everyone Feel at Home"

Dear Director:

This past Saturday, I had the opportunity to attend services with a friend who is a patient at Mount Sinai. I truly enjoyed Rabbi Spirn, the warmth of the service, and the *kiddush* that was served afterward.

Rabbi Spirn certainly makes everyone feel at home, which, I'm sure, offers great comfort to the patients and their families. Mount Sinai should be complimented for providing such a wonderful service for its patients.

Sincerely yours,

The Pull of Judaism

She had come from Russia and worked at our hospital. On many Saturday mornings, she attended our services. For Passover, she requested to borrow fifteen Haggada booklets for her Seder. She promptly returned them to me as soon as the holiday was over. Then, on her own, she asked that I recommend someone to make her kitchen kosher. She had strong feelings about her Jewish identity, and I helped her in this important decision. Though born and bred under the Communist regime, she felt the pull of Judaism.

Helping a Distinguished Rabbinical Couple

The rabbi of a prominent yeshiva planned on conducting the Passover Sedarim at the bedside of his wife, who had just been transferred from our Coronary Care Unit to a semiprivate room. His disciples called on me for help. Obviously, for a Rabbi to go through the prolonged Seder ritual while the wife's roommate entertains visitors would be an imposition on both patients. Therefore, I approached Central Listing for a single room and checked with the rebbitzin's physician to obtain permission to have her transferred. Importantly, that room had a refrigerator, which allowed the rabbi to store away homemade kosher for Passover food for three days (Saturday preceding the holiday, plus the first two days of Passover). It also had a cot brought in for the rabbi. This arrangement proved to be a real blessing as husband and wife were able to be together – instead of him having to sleep over somewhere in the neighborhood. I am very glad to say that this plan worked out beautifully. Being hospitalized on Passover is not ideal for anyone, least of all a scholar and his wife, but being together during this beautiful holiday helped maintain the spirit of Passover and gave great comfort to this rabbinical couple.

"This Sabbath Candelabrum Brought Me Luck – I Want It"

When I visited with her, we had a fine conversation. Then, when I suggested that she light a candelabrum for the Sabbath, she accepted – but only hesitatingly. When I saw her a few days later, she told me that the chemotherapy had gone off very well and that she thought that her performance of a good deed (mitzvah) for the Sabbath brought her God's help. And so, she added, she wanted permission to take this candelabrum home for use on the Sabbath and holidays. The fact is that we *lend* our patients candelabra for use while they are in the hospital. However, since this candelabrum meant so much to her, I allowed her to take it home. She, in turn, refunded me the price of another one for use inside the hospital.

Prays on the Phone

This patient requested that I return his call. When I did, he picked up his receiver, and all I heard was the recitation of the Hebrew text of Grace After Meals! Of course, that meant he was not allowed to interrupt his prayer. After he completed it, we had a good conversation in which I also congratulated him for being so diligent in religious observance.

Diminishing a Patient's Suffering

The City College
of
The City University of New York
New York, N.Y. 10031
Department of Economics
13 October 1996

Dear Rabbi Spirn:

During my stay at the Mount Sinai Medical Center (28 September–9 October 1996) I came to appreciate the highly significant role you play in diminishing a patient's suffering. Your visits, prayers, and thoughtful words of encouragement strengthened my hope and sustained my courage. Your daily lulav and ethrog reminded me of the joy I would await in the world outside the sickroom. Your profound spirituality contributed to my recovery.

What a great inspiration you are to those touched by you! The enclosed check is a small token of my gratitude. May you be spared to continue your holy work for many years to come.

Respectfully,

Professor of Economics

Enclosed: $50

Seder: Delightful...Impressive...Meaningful

April 24, 1996

Dear Director:

It is with great pleasure that I want to inform you about my delightful enjoyment at The Mount Sinai Hospital last Seder.

I was very impressed by the way Rabbi Spirn conducted the ceremony. It was very interesting to listen to him when he introduced the painful history of the Jews during the generations while explaining some sections of the Haggadah. The Talmudic interpretations mentioned by the rabbi added also meaningful insights into the Seder story.

In short, the Seder was for me a wonderful experience.

Sincerely,

Professor of Chemistry

Message from Director to Rabbi Spirn

May 6, 1996

Dr. Rabbi Spirn:

I am delighted to forward the attached (above) letter from a patient who was hospitalized at Mount Sinai this past Seder. I am pleased with the hospital's ability to attend to our patients' spiritual needs as well as physical ones. Your years of experience and dedication are valued assets which are appreciated both by the hospital and the Jewish community.

Sincerely,

Director

The Artist as a Patient

He was a painter and sculptor, and this was the first time in his life that he was hospitalized. As an outdoorsman who loved long walks, golfing, and other sports, he found time weighing heavily upon him. Being confined in a hospital room got him depressed. I spent time with him, listening to his problem. As he became more relaxed, he opened a big folder and showed me paintings he had done in his room. They were all cheerful colors, all containing flowers to a greater or lesser degree. I admired the beauty of his art and told him that he should feel quite happy while contemplating his work. Moreover, I told him, he projected life, cheer, and beauty on canvas, which means that inside himself he sensed those qualities. That surely showed a cheerful person. So why not let the inward cheerful expression of his art influence him and give him outward cheer? I told him that one view of God's occupation on His day of rest – the Sabbath – is that He contemplates the beauty of His creation!

The artist can surely imitate the Divine Creator and contemplate what he has done. "You gave me something to think about. It won't be lost," he said in parting. I returned on an extra visit a couple of days later and found him relaxed and at peace with himself.

Sabbath and Hanukkah at Our Hospital

Dear Director:

Permit me the privilege of complimenting you on your choice of our Jewish chaplain in your fine hospital.

I have spent a month and then six weeks most recently in your hospital.

Rabbi Spirn was most kind to me as he was to so many of the other patients. His Sabbath services were most inspiring and his sermons excellent. The kiddush added much to the meaning of the holiday. Having a blessing made especially for "you" at the Torah was indeed most meaningful.

I was also in the hospital for the Hanukkah party which was the nicest I have ever attended.

Rabbi Charles A. Spirn as head chaplain is doing a magnificent job. May you always continue to serve your patients so well.

With personal thanks, I remain,

Sincerely yours,

"Lovely Sabbath Service"

Dear Rabbi Spirn:

Just a token of my appreciation for the lovely Sabbath service you performed at Mount Sinai two weeks ago, and the visits you made to my room. I thank you for your kindness.

Sincerely,

Enclosed: $100

Note from Rabbi Spirn:

In the course of the year, many unsolicited donations are sent to the hospital or to me as expressions of extra gratitude for the chaplain's ministrations. They are all handed over to the administration, which deposits them in a special bank account called The Mount Sinai Jewish Chaplaincy Fund and are used for Jewish religious material. The donors receive an official receipt for their gift.

Helping Religious Outpatient

She was an outpatient, scheduled for vocal cord surgery on a Friday morning in our Short Stay Unit. She was a schoolteacher and needed reduced talking for ten days – so the end of December school vacation was just ideal for her. However, two days before her scheduled operation, she was told that it had been moved to 2:00 P.M. Her objection that the new schedule would not allow her to be home before 4:15 P.M., when the Sabbath would begin, was met with response that God would forgive her. In utter despair, she called upon me to intervene. I did and, due to the help of the clinical supervisor of the Short Stay Unit to whom I turned, the surgery was rescheduled for Friday morning at 9:00 A.M.; the patient had to be in the Unit at 7:30 A.M. Further checking indicated that everything went well, and the patient returned home in time for the beginning of the Sabbath.

A First for a Russian Jew

He was the tenth man helping us to have a quorum (*minyan*) at a Saturday morning service. Therefore, I decided to give him the honor of being called up to the Torah (an *aliyah*). He was Russian and had no Jewish education and could not recite the two special blessings: one before I read part of the weekly portion (*sidra*) from the Torah Scroll, and one after it. Foreseeing such an eventuality, I had acquired a Russian transliteration of the two Hebrew blessings and let him read from it. Indeed, it was a special experience for him, and he relished it.

"Hanukkah Party Brings So Much Joy"

Dear Rabbi,

Each year the Hanukkah party brings so much joy to so many people in the hospital. This year was no exception. We are so glad that we have been able to participate too.

We so enjoyed the cantor's singing. He was inspiring as well as most enjoyable. He was a joy to listen to and watch.

You were right. The bowl I won is beautiful. We are enjoying it very much.

The people responsible for arranging the party do a wonderful job. Please remember me to your good wife.

Most sincerely,

No Discharge on Sabbath

I had seen her a number of times in her room and at our religious services, when, on an autumn Friday afternoon, her daughter called. This woman angrily informed me that the hospital wanted her mother to be discharged on Saturday morning, the Jewish Sabbath, although her mother was a very religious person who would not violate the Sabbath. My first thought was to have her mother's physician intervene. When I called him up at this family's insistence, he replied that the decision was not in his hands but in the office of the hospital's Discharge Management. I contacted that office immediately and asked to speak to its director. Following my explanation, they graciously consented to have the patient remain here throughout the Sabbath.

Praiseworthy but Not Recommended

We live in a time when the percentage of broken marriages is high. It is comforting and admirable, therefore, to witness the profound devotion of a couple to each other. The case I ran into involved a Hassidic man who was a patient in our hospital. His wife felt that she ought to spend the Sabbath on a chair near his bed and sleep on a bench in the TV lounge of the floor in order to provide him with emotional support. One look at his wife convinced me that this plan would be detrimental to her health: She was pregnant. To persuade her to go home for the Sabbath, I stressed that her presence would increase worry and anxiety in her husband and accomplish just the reverse of what she intended. "Your husband," I told her, "would aggravate himself no end seeing you exhausting yourself on a chair for twenty-five hours and submitting your unborn child to such an ordeal. Please, listen to me: Go home, take good care of yourself, and relax during the holy Sabbath. Remember, you have an additional responsibility for the life of the fetus. Don't take risks." She listened to me, and when I saw the husband a few days later, he thanked me for my concern, which he shared. Though we admire the wife's devotion, going to such extremes must surely be discouraged.

Troubled by a Dream

At the conclusion of our Sabbath morning services, this patient approached me about a dream that troubled him immensely. In that dream, an angel told him to share his soul with his roommate. But, by doing so, the patient continued, he would die. Was the dream a prediction about his impending death? In response, I told him that the Bible (Proverbs 20:27) compares the soul to a flame. When you let someone share a flame, your flame is not extinguished and the glow is not even diminished; similarly, letting someone share your soul does not extinguish your soul but lets it remain as it was. As our patient gained peace of mind and, indeed, peace of soul, I added that the dream suggests he speak kindly to his roommate, lift up his spirits, help him be comfortable, and pray for his recovery.

A Chorus of Thank Yous

I always try to make the religious service and sermon inspiring, uplifting, and educational, and our patients are very grateful. That Saturday morning, I had an unusual experience: A dozen people attended, and when the service was completed, everyone shouted out, "Thank you! Thank you very much!" to me. Indeed, we not only worship and teach but also touch the hearts of our patients, bringing them comfort, which they appreciate fully. What greater reward can one possibly have?

A Nurse's Request

As I left the room of a patient, his private nurse followed me into the hall and asked me to please say a prayer for her as she has a difficult problem at home. I obliged and brought some relief to this nurse.

"I Want a Jewish Burial"

He was a Russian Jew who had lost most of his family in the Holocaust. We could communicate with him mainly in Yiddish, and the social worker requested that I translate. He felt he was going to die soon at our hospital and wanted to make sure he would have a Jewish burial. To calm his fears, I gave his nurse the name and phone number of the Hebrew Free Burial Society and also gave him a copy with the same information. Then, with his social worker, a plan was worked out for getting assistance in his household, to which he was soon to return. He was not critically ill, just partially incapacitated, and we prepared him for life and home.

Why Not Travel Back Home on Saturday?

A nurse from our maternity ward was puzzled by an occurrence in her unit.

A Hassidic man brought his pregnant wife over on Saturday morning, the Jewish Sabbath, in a taxi. It turned out to be a false alarm, and the prospective mother was told she might return home for a few more days. However, she declined to travel home till nightfall. The nurse could not understand why this woman was allowed to come by taxi yet could not return home the same way. The answer, of course, is that religious law allows her to violate the Sabbath when her life is in danger and that means that she was permitted to take a taxi to the hospital. Returning home, however, was no longer a matter of danger to life, and, therefore, the law of the Sabbath is fully applicable to her, and she may not ride a car. I told the nurse to get her a kosher meal and let her remain on our premises till nightfall, when the Sabbath ends.

Setting up the Lighting of Sabbath Candelabra

A student at the Jewish Theological Seminary, who serves as the Jewish chaplain at Our Lady of Mercy Hospital in the Bronx, was directed to me for information on how to set up a service for the lighting of the Sabbath lights by Jewish women patients. I was glad to share the concept of electric Sabbath candelabra. I told him where to buy them, how to attach laminated cards with the blessings, and how to organize the delivery and retrieval of such candelabra. I also sent him samples of our literature on this subject. Subsequently, in a letter to me, he writes: "The candelabra were far more beautiful than I ever expected and meant so much to my patients during the Holy Day season. They will continue to be used throughout the year, of course. I now want to thank you for your excellent suggestions."

Not Religious?

As I identified myself to this patient, he quickly responded that he was not religious. However, as I talked to him about his health, he grew friendlier. As I was about to leave, he called me back and said, "Do you have any 'pull' upstairs? Put in a prayer for me."

5: FAMILY PROBLEMS

Problems During Pregnancy

Every so often, we find young women on our maternity floors who have encountered problems during their pregnancy and have, therefore, become long-term patients of ours. The question then is how to prevent them from falling into a depression at worst or, at best, being fearful, anxious patients.

I usually make it a point to see such patients at least twice or three times a week after I had talked to them, striving to increase their peace of mind, improve their self-image and their self-confidence.

- First, I tell such a woman: It is not your fault. I see women like you very often in our maternity ward, and, therefore, it is a general problem, and you are not the only one who has it.
- Being in a hospital should give you and your husband and family a great deal of peace of mind rather than distress. Here you will get immediate help in case of need, so please relax.
- What is more: While you are not allowed to be very active physically, intellectually your mind is free. So spend your time catching up on your reading, watching TV programs, listening to the radio or tapes that you enjoy.
- Do not overlook the problems you do not have. Think of it: You *have* conceived a child. You and your husband do not have to spend months searching for a child to adopt, spending many thousands of dollars, struggling with a foreign government to get an exit visa for the child and then traveling to Romania, Cambodia, or China, etc.
- You feel somewhat isolated? Well, the telephone has already been invented. You can easily be in touch with those you care for and who care about you. And, of course, you are welcome to have visitors.
- I like to tell about a young mother who, during her fourth pregnancy, encountered problems and stayed here for three months, after which she introduced her newborn daughter to me. No depression and no complaints. She left as a happy mother, and so can you.

- Today is Friday. I like to invite you to light our Sabbath electric candelabrum a half-hour before sunset. After you recite the blessing on the card which I am giving you, I recommend something more. The moment of the lighting of candles is as important as Yom Kippur. So after the blessing over the lights, do offer a special personal prayer to God. You may say: "Dear God, please grant me two wishes: a healthy child and that the birth comes at the right time. And please, dear God, keep me well."
- Another important point: Remember that you are here because you want to protect your infant. When the baby grows up, you will be able to tell him or her how much you loved your child even before birth.
- As a final point, I want to give you a special card as extra protection (*Segulah*). I am not a Hassid, but the Lubavitcher Rebbe, of blessed memory, was a great and saintly man. Through his ladies' organization, he sent me these cards with the proviso that I give one to any Jewish woman who encounters problems during pregnancy. On it is Psalm 121: "I lift up my eyes to the mountains, from where shall my help come? My help comes from the Lord who made heaven and earth." He also added Jewish mystical symbols on the card. Protect the card in an envelope or a napkin, as God's name is on it, and place it under your pillow.

Some of these may help her through reassurance, others give her a chance to do something active to promote her own well-being. I thus lift the spirit of the worrying maternity patient. As one social worker who observed me in action said to me later: "Rabbi, you have left a changed person." This concern and guidance fosters hope and trust in God when the patient needs it most and often results in tangible improvement in the patient's mood and outlook.

Abandoned Child

In Pediatrics, I noticed a three-and-a-half-year-old child calling a nurse "Mommy." Upon inquiry, it turned out that this infant was Jewish but had been abandoned and raised by a Catholic foster home for children that sent him to our hospital for treatment. Following contact with the Social Service of our hospital and of the Catholic foster home, the fact emerged that the child was born out of wedlock to a Jewish woman described as "less than balanced," who had intermarried in the meantime and refused to accept her sickly son. I then contacted the Jewish Child Care Association which, with the approval of the Catholic foster home, has promised to place this child in a Jewish foster home.

Maternity Patient and Hannah's Prayer

Her room in our maternity unit was filled with vases of flowers, and she was full of smiles and very happy. We do expect that on the maternity floors. But in this case, it was an overabundance and an overflowing of joy and self-contentment. Reason? She had been childless for six years of marriage and had yearned for a baby. And God had now heard her prayer and blessed her with a daughter.

"Do you remember the first chapter in I Samuel wherein Hannah pours out her heart to God for a child? And then how grateful she is in the second chapter, after God blessed her with a son, Samuel?" I asked.

"Yes," she replied. Throughout the past years, she had read that first chapter many times. Now, she said, with the arrival of her child, she and her entire family are exceedingly happy and grateful. Now she also reads the second chapter and expresses her joy and her faith in God's work and Providence in the words of Hannah, which we also read in the synagogue as the Haftorah of the first day of Rosh Hashanah.

How beautiful to witness such appreciation of a precious gift from God!

A Surprise Request from Maternity

I wished the couple mazel tov when the husband, who was holding his newborn child, said that he and his wife were B.T.s. At the moment, I did not identify those initials, so he explained to me that they were *Baalay Teshuvah* – returnees to Judaism and Jewish observance. Then he had a question for me: where would they get help in making their kitchen kosher! I promised to contact a religious group that is very knowledgeable in the laws of *kashruth* and assists people in introducing it in their homes. As I carried out my promise, I could not help but think that one could never know who and where a Jewish person might make a move to return to Jewish tradition.

Conflict About Naming a Child

A serious conflict arose about what Hebrew name to give to a newborn child. The mother wanted to perpetuate the name of a late dear grandfather of hers. Her mother-in-law, however, was adamant about perpetuating the name of her late father whom she had loved very much and who had no other child except herself.

What ensued in the maternity ward was a quarrel between mother-in-law and daughter-in-law. Anger and tears were precipitated by that family quarrel. I was asked for a rabbinic decision. My answer was that the baby's mother should be given the privilege of having her first child named the way she wanted. Otherwise, we would also run the risk of the mother being always resentful, and some of that resentment might rub off on the child –

something we must avoid at all cost. Now, to take care of the mother-in-law's need, an understanding should be reached with the young mother that when a second child is born, the mother-in-law's father's name should be perpetuated. I further indicated that peace and love ought to prevail in the family, and all should be grateful to God that they are all celebrating a very happy event.

Artificial Insemination

I have never had to deal with this type of problem before, and so I established contact with the physicians of our hospital's In-Vitro Fertilization Unit. The case involved a religious man whose wife needed artificial insemination with the semen of her husband. The couple wanted to produce the semen in the privacy of a hotel room. It had to be done on the eve of the Sabbath, because that was at the peak of the wife's fertility. And so the problem arose of carrying the semen from the hotel to the clinic on the Sabbath, when carrying is prohibited by Jewish law. The semen had to be brought over to the clinic very promptly, since the insemination had to be performed within an hour. We resolved the problem by using the help of a non-Jewish messenger. Our prayer was that God bless this couple with a child.

Adding a Name

A young woman in her twenties was a frequent patient at our hospital. She requested the addition of a Hebrew name to the one she had, as a petition to God for healing. We did it at a Sabbath service and at our Torah Scroll in presence of her family and friends. Her condition did improve, thank Heaven.

Perform a Cesarean

The husband of a Maternity patient turned to me with an unusual question. His wife's obstetrician and another physician recommended that she undergo a Cesarean section to deliver her twins. The husband, a Sephardic Jew, wanted to find out what religious law (halakhah) would recommend. I referred him to a colleague of mine, Rabbi Moshe D. Tendler, who is the chairman of the biology department of Yeshiva University and a specialist in medical problems. Upon hearing details of this case, such as the fact that the pregnancy had completed its full term, that the mother was a little older than average and prone to high blood pressure, etc., Rabbi Tendler ruled that the Cesarean be done. This gave peace of mind to the couple. I am glad to state that mother and twins are doing well.

Bright Youngster in a Broken Home

This youngster was a patient in our department of Pediatric Psychiatry. He was a bright, handsome boy, unfortunately a victim of a broken home where chaotic fights took place. This affected his behavior in his Hebrew Day School where he became disruptive in class, found it difficult to concentrate, and threw tantrums. His mother, embarrassed by this behavior, came to me for help. She felt guilty about her son's behavior. I tried to give her support and contacted both the child's psychiatrist and the school's principal. The psychiatrist recommended the boy be placed in a very structured setting in a smaller class with greater personal attention. While the school does not at present have such a class for his grade, the principal assured me that the child is learning and will be placed in such a class the following term. With the child continuing in therapy as an outpatient and the school aware of his needs, I felt the child should not be transferred to another school. Chances for improvement seemed positive to me. A thank-you card from the mother confirmed my prognosis. It said: "Thank you so much for taking time to speak with me. Thanks also for your inquiries and intervention on my behalf. It had a very positive effect with the psychiatrist and the school's principal. Your thoughtfulness meant much more than words can ever say. I appreciate your efforts and concern."

Naming a Child After Deceased Sibling?

The father of a newborn child in our maternity ward asked this question of me. He was somewhat apprehensive to do that and wanted rabbinic guidance. In reply, I told him that this was a very legitimate question. The answer lies in adding a second name to the name of the deceased, a name that prayerfully refers to longevity and Divine Providence. This solution satisfied the father, and it put his mind at ease.

Three First Names

This Maternity patient was clearly upset after the birth of her first child, a boy. She and her husband had decided on giving the child first and middle Hebrew names when her mother-in-law pressured her to add a third name – the name of her mother. It looked almost like a series of names usually given to British royalty. Promising the mother-in-law that, in good time, when a second child arrived, that name would be used first, proved to be of no avail. She wanted it *now*. Therefore, to keep the peace of the family, I suggested translating the feminine name into a close masculine one. This child would then have three first names, or, in other words, one first name and two middle ones. Fearing conflicts about designating godparents for the ritual circumcision, this young mother also had me spell out, in detail, the entire procedure. With that in hand, she was relieved and happy.

Hospitalized Grandfather to Witness Bar-Mitzvah

Dear ---:

During the past month my father was a patient at the hospital. During his stay, through the help of Rabbi Spirn, my son was able to have a "Bar-Mitzvah service" in the chapel.

The ceremony was a very meaningful experience for me, my son, and my father, and I feel that it would not have been possible without the help of Rabbi Spirn. Therefore, as a token of our appreciation, my wife and I are contributing the enclosed $1,000 to the Mount Sinai Medical Center, to be used at the discretion of Rabbi Spirn for the chapel. Perhaps he'll be able to use it during the Passover festival.

Sincerely,

Enclosed: $1,000
CC: Rabbi Spirn

Effecting Reconciliation of Family

A member of our staff and his wife presented an interesting problem to me. A nephew of that couple was going to be confirmed (Bar-Mitzvah) in four days at Saturday morning services in their synagogue. The wife of our staff member, though invited, felt she could not attend – and her husband would not want to attend without his wife – because past grudges and lack of communication had disrupted those two families. There were tears and expressions of hurt feelings. It dawned on me that the only way to resolve this family squabble was to effectuate reconciliation. Therefore, I made an immediate call to the father of the Bar-Mitzvah candidate and urged him to meet with his brother and sister-in-law and do so *before* the Bar-Mitzvah and not after it, as he suggested to me. "We will be more than cordial," he assured me. Upon my insistence, he promised to call them the next day, which was a legal holiday. Result: he kept his promise and called them, and he and his wife met our couple in a "neutral place." After two hours of discussion, they arrived at a reconciliation. Thus the story had a happy ending – a reunited and reconciled family. "You have helped us end a three-year cold war, Rabbi," said this staff member to me after that Bar-Mitzvah. "Everything was just excellent. Thank you."

Wants Psalm 27

A patient with a cancer diagnosis requested a copy of the English translation of Psalm 27. I obliged. When he received it, his eyes immediately turned to the verse: "I have faith that I shall yet experience the goodness of the Lord in the land of the living." His eyes filled up with tears. He would so much like to see his grandson's upcoming Bar-Mitzvah. He found a measure of comfort and hope in this Psalm.

Help to Teenager

He was a nice, handsome teenager admitted to our psychiatric floor because he suffered from a mood disorder and got out of control. That led him to the Quiet Room, where a strap attached each arm and leg to his bed and a nurse remained in constant surveillance of him. He resented the restraint and clamored to be untied. I tried to calm him down by pointing out that this situation was temporary, and that the sooner he gained control over himself, the sooner he would be released. His parents too called on me, asking that I see him every day and be of help to him. It was a rough week for him. Slipping behind in his studies worried him, as did his inability to pray fully in his phylacteries (tefillin). I gave him some abbreviated prayer texts in card form and left a regular prayer book with the nursing staff to give him when safe to do so. Throughout his stay, I gave Sabbath rolls (challahs) and a bottle of the kosher grape juice Kedem to the nursing staff for safekeeping. They would give him the juice in a paper cup for Kiddush (blessing on wine) on the Sabbath. I was also in constant touch with his psychiatrist, the nursing staff, and his family, whom I guided throughout this painful experience.

I am glad to say that the young man's condition improved markedly with time and treatment. He was then allowed to use his phylacteries and attend our Sabbath services. "You have a lovely young man as your son," I said to his mother on her regular visits. In time, he recovered beautifully and went home, discharged by his physician and blessed by this chaplain.

Religiosity – Always on Same High Level?

He was a bearded young man and always wore a skullcap. He moved in a wheelchair after amputation of a leg due to an accident. He approached me at the conclusion of one Sabbath morning service, when my sermon had dealt with faith. I had related a parable with the moral that as long as some embers of faith glow in a person's heart, they can rise and burst into a bright and radiant flame of faith. This young man painfully complained that, at times, he was not in the mood to pray. He was worried about his religiosity.

I put his mind at ease by telling him that it is very normal for a human being not to be on the same high level of religious fervor at all times. Life is easy for no one, and we are not always able to pray with great intent and feeling. Judaism teaches us to carry out the law – pray even when not in the best mood for prayer. Keep up your receptivity to prayer, I told him. Then, when the mood does strike you, when you are inspired to pray, as on the High Holy Days or on special occasions, you will have the capacity to rise to a high level of feeling. You must always cultivate the sparks and then you will find that they can burst into a flame of faith, hope, comfort, and inspiration. That explanation of the spiritual life of the believing person gave this person reassurance that his faith was still strong. He left me with a smile on his face.

Muslem Mother Asks for a Mohel

In an unusual telephone call, a woman who identified herself as being of the Islamic faith inquired about a rabbi who can perform a ritual circumcision on her son. We do know that Muslims also practice circumcision. While we appreciate her confidence in a Jewish mohel, I advised her to contact her own spiritual leader, who would no doubt recommend the proper functionary. Later on, I came across a pediatric surgeon who is also a religious man, and he told me that he would perform the circumcision of a Muslim child.

Panic in Maternity

She was in panic in her maternity room, and I was called in urgently. Her baby had air in the chest cavity which pressed on the heart and on one lung, and it had been taken up to the Infant ICU, on Klingenstein Pavilion's 9th floor. The mother had had two miscarriages before and was very anxious about the survival of this child. She cried bitter tears, which relieved her somewhat. Then she said that her physician had mentioned that she should see a psychiatrist. This suggestion distressed her, since, given her past experiences, her tears were not morbid but easily understandable. What she needed was good news about her child's recovery. I helped her find hope that, with God's help, the infant would recover. She asked for prayer texts, which I brought her, and I promised to see her again the following morning. When I did, I found her relaxed and satisfied. The child's condition had improved. She was very grateful for my counseling. She quoted my statements to her and the healing effect they had had on her. When I returned a third time, she was ready to be discharged, while her child would remain a few more days for observation. She was pleased and relaxed and again thanked me profusely for pulling her through her crisis.

Bearing a First Child at Age Thirty-Five?

An unusual request was made of me from an outside caller. He wanted to know if there was any risk of bearing a child at age thirty-five. He needed that information for a friend of his who wished to build a family but whose girlfriend was that old. I checked on this matter with our Maternity Department, and was told that in most cases, everything turns out fine, but there is an increased risk of congenital defects in the fetus, which can be determined by analysis of the amniotic fluid during pregnancy. Hopefully, by the grace of God, all would turn out well in this case.

Problem About Hebrew and English Names

She had given birth to a healthy baby boy, yet I found her sitting in a chair and crying. After identifying myself and encouraging her to share her problem with me, she revealed an unusual story. She and her husband had decided to give the child the Hebrew name of her grandfather, but a different English name. However, her aged grandmother, who, she told me, was the real head of the family, insisted that the English name, too, be exactly that of her late husband. An irreconcilable conflict ensued, making our patient miserable. My suggestion was to tell her grandmother always to call the child by the Hebrew name, which was that of her husband, and also to assure her that, in her presence, the parents of the child would also call him by his Hebrew name. That should assuage her feelings and, being a matriarch, make her feel proud that the Hebrew name is being continued. Moreover, the English name decided on by the parents had some connection with Hanukkah, during which the child was born, and that should count too. The mother cheered up, and I left her with the advice not to argue with her grandmother, but only to humor her and treat her with diplomacy.

The *Gomel* Prayer

The questioner, an employee of our hospital, called to inquire about the special prayer one is to recite upon escape from danger. Her boyfriend had escaped unscathed from a mugging experience. The answer was that he is to be called up to the Torah during a prayer service and recite the *Gomel* blessing, thanking God for having saved his life.

Cesarean Birth: When Is Circumcision Done?

Among the many questions that occur in a hospital was the following: A baby boy was born on Friday night by Cesarean section. Is it permissible to have his ritual circumcision on the eighth day, which comes on a Saturday? Answer: In such a case, the circumcision is to be performed on the ninth day – a Sunday.

Selection of Godparents at Circumcision – No Problem

This young mother in our maternity ward was upset by family bickering over who should be the godparents (*Kvater*) at the ritual circumcision of her son. She turned to me for help. In response, I gave her the details on how to arrange the ceremony so as to include all the contenders. Her agitation gave way to a smile of happiness.

A Physician and a Good Mohel: Both Qualified

A physician at a Brooklyn hospital called to request a physician who is also a practicing mohel to perform the circumcision on his newborn son. Luckily, I know of such a physician who is also qualified both religiously and surgically. At the same time, I also informed him that the official mohel at our hospital, though not a physician, has been surgically trained here, is fully religious, and is highly competent and qualified. I gave him both names and received profound thanks in turn.

Father and Son – Same First Name?

A patient in our maternity ward asked whether it was permissible to name her newborn son with the same first name as his father. The answer is that it is contrary to the practice and tradition of Ashkenazic Jews to name a child after a living person. I then offered her alternative suggestions, one of which she just loved.

Compassion of a Physician at Death of Infant

The infant son of an Israeli couple on an education mission to this country developed a serious illness – leukemia – which, after three months of treatment at our Pediatric Unit, became terminal when pneumonia set in. At midnight on a Saturday night, one of the child's physicians had me contacted, asking to call her back at her home in New Jersey. She was deeply worried about how the family would take this tragedy. I reassured her after seeing the father of the child. On Sunday morning, as I visited the family again, the child had died, and plans were being made for a funeral service in Brooklyn and then flying to Israel for burial. As I stood with the family, the physician arrived from New Jersey. She enveloped the mother of the child in a tender embrace, and they cried together in each other's arms. Indeed, the physician had become close to the family and completely identified with the tragedy of the loss of the child. This display of sympathy and shared grief pointed up the profound humanity of this professional. I stayed on for two and a half hours, as did the physician, till the funeral director arrived and then walked with the tearful family to the hearse, while the funeral director carried the child's body in his arms. We intoned Psalm 91 and the verse, "They shall hold you in their hands to keep you from hurting" was reality, sad reality.

I had offered words of support and consolation to the family and, of course, to this most compassionate doctor, as I too strongly felt the impact of this tragedy. How surprised and moved I was when a few years later, I received the following missive:

"A Lifelong Impact"

Dear Rabbi Spirn:

You and I met a number of years ago while I was in training. My fellowship in pediatric hematology-oncology took place at Mount Sinai between 1984 and 1986. One dawn toward the latter part of that time I lost a patient to whom I had become extremely attached. I think that for many physicians during training there is a crucial turning point experience. Having sat at Moshie's bedside all night, hoping against hope that he would make it, using whatever medical know-how we had to pull him through – and failing –was the most daunting, disappointing experience I had ever had. I cannot tell you what a major role you played, with your words of comfort not only to the family but also to me as a young physician in turning that very negative experience into a "life-building" experience.

I am in practice as a pediatric hematologist-oncologist for seven years now in a university hospital setting. I have seen many times of joy and times of grief among the families of my patients as well as among the residents and students that care for them. I will never forget in my dealings with them what my experience with you at Moshie's bedside taught me. Just a few words of encouragement and consolation will have a lifelong impact. After all these years I'd like to say thank you.

---, M.D.
Assistant Professor Pediatrics
Division of Hema/Oncology
University of Miami
School of Medicine

December 25 – Bar-Mitzvah at Our Hospital

An unusual event took place at our hospital on Thursday morning, December 25, 1986: a Bar-Mitzvah ceremony. The young man was thirteen, which is the age for a Bar-Mitzvah, and he was going to be confirmed formally two days later on a Saturday morning in his family's synagogue. What brought him and his family and friends – some twenty-five people – to take part in the full Thursday service in the Patients' Lounge of Guggenheim 6 was that he wanted his dear grandfather, a terminal patient on that floor, to witness and participate in the ceremony of attaining religious responsibility. I am glad to record that our hospital staff fully cooperated with us by not only allowing us to use the lounge but also extending itself in numerous ways in order to make the event possible and as festive as could be. The patient was wheeled in from his room and received the honor of being called up to the Torah (aliyah). The Scroll was the one we use for our regular Sabbath services. It was a very moving ceremony with the patient's physician standing behind to watch him as he offered the prayer at the Torah. At the request of the family, I delivered a brief sermon fitting the occasion, as did the father of the young man. A most devoted member of our nursing staff kept checking that all tubes feeding medication to our patient were in place.

The son-in-law of our patient wrote me as follows:

> I want to thank you on behalf of my entire family for your work in organizing a special Bar-Mitzvah service for my father-in-law. Although the entire weekend was a thrill of all of us, this particular service – Thursday morning – was something special and in a certain way the high point. For my father-in-law, it meant everything in the world. Even my mother-in-law, who felt torn by our plans for a simhah [celebration] for our son's Bar-Mitzvah, found the Thursday davening [prayer service] as an unexpected and wonderful way of having my father-in-law included in the Bar-Mitzvah.
>
> Indeed, it was the will to participate in his grandson's Bar-Mitzvah that enabled the grandfather to extend his life span. Exactly two weeks later, he returned his soul to his Divine Maker. The Bar-Mitzvah had thus become the apex of his life in this world.

Terrified Patient

Her nurse called me to visit the literally terrified patient who had a serious problem. She had just been told that she had a malignant rectal tumor. "I am scared stiff," she told me. "I don't want to die." I let her unburden herself and voice her fears. Her physician suggested radiation. After talking for a while, she became a little more relaxed. I suggested to her a three-pronged plan. First: to accept the oncologist's treatment. Second: not to spoil the present time for herself and her husband (she had no children) because of possible future problems but do her best to function now as well as possible. Third: prayer, asking God for help and prolongation of her life. I saw her three days in succession. Then she told me the physician recommended she become an outpatient in our radiation clinic. I left her a little more at peace with herself and on her way home.

Guiding a Maternity Patient to Peace of Mind

She was twenty-eight weeks pregnant with her third child when she started bleeding and having other symptoms that resulted in her hospitalization. Our physicians did not allow her to get out of bed for eight weeks. This affected her very strongly. Being confined to bed and worrying constantly about herself and the life of her fetus proved unbearable to her. She became tearful and alarmist. I visited her a few times every week, and in addition, she called frequently and asked for immediate visits. During my visits, which could last for a full hour, she listened carefully and then, taking a notebook from her night table, often asked me to dictate to her my conversation and uplifting words so that, when she felt low in spirit and worrisome, she could read what I had said and regain a sense of balance and hope. At the end of the eight weeks, she was permitted to go home. Two weeks later, on her thirty-eighth week, she returned to our hospital and gave birth to a perfectly normal and healthy baby boy.

6: PERSONAL PROBLEMS

Yael – Israeli War Orphan – at Our Hospital

In the 1973 Yom Kippur War in Israel, a pilot was killed and a fellow pilot married the widow and adopted her orphaned infant child, Yael. In 1988, the child, at the age of fifteen, developed cancer of the knees. The couple found out that a noted American specialist at our hospital would be the best surgeon for Yael. When I entered their room during one of my regular visits to the Falk Adolescent Pavilion, I found the family in despair, with the mother crying uncontrollably and, identifying me, clamored: "Help, Rabbi, help."

What happened? This is what I was told: Being of modest means, Yael's stepfather had gone to then Defense Minister Yitzchak Rabin, who immediately offered financial help from Israel's defense budget to cover the family's trip to America and the approximate cost of the surgery. By now, Yael had already had one operation. However, the surgeon felt she needed a second operation – but the family lacked the additional funds and was in despair. Saving the child was on their minds and, yes, it was on mine too.

So instinctively and intuitively, I asked the mother to please stop crying and stay with the child while I asked the stepfather to follow me. I took him to the office of the hospital director and told the secretary I needed an urgent appointment, which was granted to me. To start a conversation, I began by telling the director that a mazel tov was due to me as I had just performed the wedding of my daughter. He shook my hand. Then I quoted to him a passage of the Talmud in English: "He who has mercy on others, God has mercy on him." He grasped my point quickly and asked, "What do you request?"

I told him the story of the pilot who married the widow of a fellow pilot and adopted her infant child, now fifteen, and gravely ill at our hospital. I also told him of Rabin's immediate response in extending financial help to the war orphan, but it was not enough to cover a second surgery. I requested mercy and heroism. In response, the director agreed to cover all hospital charges for Yael. An application had to be filled out. I wrote on it,

"Confidential and Urgent." The pilot had witnessed my conversation with the director and expressed our deepest gratitude to him.

When we returned to the child's room and told his wife the story, she burst out in tears, tears of joy this time, and wanted to thank me. She asked what she could do for me, and I answered that there was no need for her to do anything for me, but I made two recommendations: try to light the Sabbath candles and to make an effort to eat kosher. I blessed the child and wished her well.

P.S. Yael went home before Rosh Hashanah and was walking on her own two feet.

Overidentification with Jewish Suffering

Dear Rabbi Spirn:

I am writing to wish you belated Hanukkah greetings, as well as best wishes for a happy, healthy and prosperous New Year. As a patient who was under your jurisdiction – I could even say "care" – at Mount Sinai, I wanted to say hello and to let you know how much you helped me and how often I think of, and derive strength from, some of the things that you told me in our talks together.

You may remember me as the girl who had recently been studying Jewish History, and was very disturbed by certain aspects of the Holocaust. I came to your Saturday services and could not stop crying. You told me: "Young lady, you will recover completely."

Rabbi Spirn, indeed I did. I left the hospital after a very short time. I have not been seriously ill since then, and for that I can only pray and give thanks.

It meant a lot to me to have a visitor such as you, and to be able to talk about a few of the things that were bothering me then. Whenever things seem too hopeless, I remember what you said: "Do you think I don't have my arguments with God too?" Thank you for your willingness to spend so much time with me and for your faith in me. I can honestly say that you helped me as much, if not more, than the doctors. May you be spared the strength to continue your aid and comfort to those who suffer.

All the best to you and your family for the New Year,

Sincerely,

The Supervisor of the Hospital's Chaplaincy Program

Dear Rabbi Spirn:

This acknowledges the receipt of a letter of commendation from a former patient.

It is gratifying to know that your efforts on behalf of the patients are recognized and acknowledged.

It is certainly true that we never know the extent of our influence upon the lives of others. It is reminiscent of the ripples which result from a stone tossed into a pond – where those ripples touch is never known!

With best wishes for continued success during the New Year.

Sincerely,

Recommending a Doctor for a Second Opinion

Dear Director:

I would like to take this opportunity to praise Rabbi Dr. Charles A. Spirn, head chaplain, for the outstanding effort he made during my stay at Mount Sinai Hospital.

I had a partial hysterectomy with a large fibroid tumor removed on January 31, 1985. During the next several days, I developed several complications that caused me to be in serious pain.

Rabbi Spirn visited me during my second week in the hospital, and saw my anguish and pain. He took the time to find out what my problems were, and insisted on calling my doctor to inquire of my continuing pain and suffering with hope to resolve my problem. The next morning I called Rabbi Spirn, since I was still in pain, to ask him to please recommend a urologist to come in on my case. I called my doctor, and the doctor the rabbi recommended with my doctor's permission was brought in on the case that afternoon.

He changed the method of treatment, and my pain and suffering was gradually alleviated. I was finally well enough to go home with medication on February 18, 1985. It should be noted that Rabbi Spirn followed up on my case. My own doctor was grateful and praised the rabbi for being concerned and alerting him to my needs.

In reviewing my stay at Mount Sinai Hospital, I feel that the turning point in my recovery was the compassion and ability of this rabbi to take action. This rabbi didn't come in and say "God bless you" and "Goodbye," but tried to help me where it really counted.

Every hospital should have a Rabbi Dr. Charles A. Spirn to look after the real needs of the sick and helpless.

Yours truly,

A Rabbi, Professor, and National Leader

His letter to president of the New York Board of Rabbis:

Dear Rabbi ---:

It has been well said that in times of stress laymen can turn to rabbis, but rabbis generally have no rabbis to turn to. All of us who have tried to help the ill, whether as chaplains or through individual visitations, know how welcome our efforts are.

This past August I had the opportunity of learning this truth from the patient's angle. Because of some surgical procedures, I had to spend three weeks at Mount Sinai Hospital. During my stay, the chaplain of the hospital, Rabbi Spirn, visited me regularly in the course of his work. His genuine concern, his warm friendliness, and his quiet sense of hope did a great deal to buoy my spirits and sustain my faith during the long ordeal.

Thank God, the prayers of family and friends have been answered, and I am now completing the process of recuperation at home. I shall always cherish the memory of Rabbi Spirn's presence during this period.

Sincerely,
Rabbi ---

CC: Rabbi Spirn

A Paradoxical Intervention*

A psychiatrist called to solicit my help. He wanted my intervention in making a twenty-five to thirty-year-old patient in our psychiatric unit eat his meals, which he was stubbornly refusing to do. The question in my mind was: How do you do that? Just having a rabbi urge him to have his meal, it seemed to me, would get us nowhere. He had already heard that from his dietician, his male nurse, and his physician.

As I reached his floor, I found that the patient, who wore a beard, was sitting motionless at a table in a lounge, with an unopened tray in front of him. I introduced myself as an Orthodox rabbi, greeted him and sat down

---

*From Rabbi Spirn's article in the *Jewish Chaplain*, Winter 1996, Magazine of the National Association of Jewish Chaplains, published by permission.

opposite him. He watched me as I examined the tray and its label carefully and then firmly declared that this was a kosher meal but that he was not to touch it. The idea came to me to play it his way, encouraging him not to eat, since that was his attitude. This way, too, I would avoid a no answer to me.

The solution – it appeared to me – after gaining his confidence, was to shift eventually to statements about religion to which, as a pious person, he could not say no. "This tray has kosher food all right," I told him, "but you are not allowed to eat it. Don't you know that a religious Jew, a *ben Torah*, must first wash his hands?" Surprisingly, he answered that he could not wash his hands because he could not get a cup at the sink.

"Well," I said to him, "I will find a cup for you. Come with me to the sink." At that invitation, he stood up and followed me to the sink, where I got him a cup of water, poured it on his hands and told him to repeat after me the Hebrew blessing of *Al Netilas Yadayim*. He, of course, did repeat the blessing. Then, as we walked back to his seat, I told him he may not talk after that blessing. I then promptly opened the tray, took the bread from it and told him to recite the blessing on bread in a loud, clear voice. "Repeat after me: *Boruch*..." After this blessing, one *must* eat some bread. So he did it automatically and took a bite. As he looked at me, I carefully examined all the foods on the tray and told him they were strictly kosher. Then, taking the cutlery, I cut some of the meat and gave it to him on a fork. He took it and, with my encouragement, yes, he ate the full meal. "It is not finished yet," I continued. "The law is you have to *bentch* [to say the Grace After Meals]. If you know it well by heart – fine. Otherwise, I will help you. We must do what the Torah requires." And so, with some help from me, he recited the full text of the Grace. I then congratulated him for carrying out religious requirements and praised him for being a truly religious Jew.

Thus, through my paradoxical intervention, telling the pious patient the opposite of what I really wanted him to do, I overcame his refusal to eat. By directing my efforts not directly toward eating and risking a rebuff, but toward religious requirements to which, as a fully religious person, he could not say no, I resolved the psychiatrist's dilemma. As his male nurse who had watched my successful intervention from a distance approached us and saw an empty tray and a satisfied patient, he exclaimed: "You surely have the right words, Rabbi."

Message to Amputee: "No Detour Please"

We recurrently have cases of leg amputation in our hospital. Its effect on the patient can be traumatic indeed. Visitations, counseling and praying by the chaplain are self-understood and enable the patient to face surgery. What about after surgery? How do you make such a person readjust to life and ignite his will to live and not to fall apart? Based on my experience at our hospital, I tell the amputee:

"You have done well. Your surgery was successful. Be grateful for that. Now, the hospital will adjust an artificial leg to you and teach you to walk by yourself or to move in an electric wheelchair. Of course, it is best to have the use of one's own legs. But under the circumstances, you will still be able to function well. You have been blessed with a loving family to whom you will be able to continue to relate, and you will also be able to pursue your profession without much hindrance. Please count the blessings you do have. They are substantial. If, however, you let yourself drift into self-pity and depression, then you will create for yourself a psychological problem, which may require hospitalization in psychiatry, and then you will be right back where you were before: with the artificial leg. I had such a case in our hospital involving a physician, a member of the community where I had served as a rabbi, and it pained me very much when I found him later in psychiatry. Luckily, he recovered quickly.

"So, my dear friend, what do you need the detour to psychiatry for? Get hold of your emotions now, make up your mind that you will accept yourself as you are now and do your best to lead as normal a life as possible. Your physical condition is involuntary and beyond your control. But in your psychological reaction to the new situation, you have much control. So don't you voluntarily let yourself drift into a depression. In the language of religion: learn to live with it and use your reserves of accumulated faith and your willpower to steer yourself to life and personal and professional fulfillment. You have it within yourself. I recommend that you use it now and in the future. God give you a long and happy life."

My guidance had a positive effect on this highly educated patient and his devoted wife who had listened to my talk. Yes, he did return to his professional career for many years and kept me informed about his activities.

"Rabbi, What Do You Do with So Many Mitzvoth?"

It was in the afternoon of Rosh Hashanah when I accompanied the wife of a very seriously ill patient in our Cardiac CU. There we met friends of that family, who had come to inquire about the patient's state of health. Seeing me active at the hospital and, what is more, on a major Holy Day, one of their nonreligious friends was amazed at my extending myself beyond the call of duty and inquisitively asked, "Rabbi, what do you do with so many mitzvoth?" Well, I answered him, I keep them in reserve in God's Mitzvah Deposit. And I pray to God that He be merciful and gracious (*rachum ve chanun*) to me and enable me to continue bringing comfort and hope – and a measure of faith – to those I am called upon to minister. I further pray that

God answer my prayers for patients and pull them through to life and recovery.

"I Need Emotional Support"

I found the following message on my voice mail: "I need emotional support. Can you come to see me?"

When I entered her room, the young woman was in a mood of despair. She had persistent headaches and feared the worst. Tests were scheduled for the next day but how can one wait till the next day? Her situation brought to mind a poem by the French romantic poet Alfred de Musset: "I need a prayer to survive till next day." After some conversation, I invited her to recite a prayer that I presented to her. As she read it aloud, she burst out crying. The prayer expressed well in words what was in her heart. As she continued reading it, she regained her composure and a degree of confidence and trust that God heard her prayer and would help her. The text follows:

Our Father, our King! Send a perfect healing to the sick of Thy people. Send me, O God, Thy healing, that I may speedily recover from the illness that has come upon me. Sustain my spirit, relieve my pain, and restore me to perfect health, happiness, and usefulness. Instill in my body Thy healing balm that I may continue to be able to bear testimony to Thy everlasting mercy and love, for Thou O Lord, art a faithful and merciful healer. Amen.

We talked some more. Then I offered a formal prayer for recovery, which included her Hebrew name. I also promised to include her in my private devotions.

Plea to a Physician: Treat the Person

He was terminally ill and his devoted wife spent whole days in his room. The physician had prescribed treatment. Yet what this couple requested insistently was seeing the physician, which could give the patient the courage to go on and lift his spirits.

I called the physician's office and left a message saying that I felt his visit would mean a lot to the patient. A half-hour later, as I walked in the halls of our hospital, whom do I meet? Yes, that very physician. I know him very well and have a very high regard for him. He also happens to be a very religious man. And so I told him that I was sure that he offered his prayers to God that morning. One of the prayers, however, refers to God as the "Competent and Merciful Healer (*Rofay Neemon Verachamon*)," with the implication that we, especially human physicians, are to imitate this Divine attribute – we call that *Imitatio Dei*. "Judaism requests that we not only treat the illness but also the person. And this person needs your presence, your compassion.

Please see him now." The physician promised to do so. True, he had visited this patient often enough, but would see him again now, to bring mental and emotional support to a very sick patient.

My message to all doctors is: Imitate the Divine Healer. Exercise not only your competence, but also your humanity and compassion, when your patients need you.

Charters Plane to Go to The Mount Sinai Hospital

This elderly gentleman became sick during his vacation in New Hampshire and was hospitalized there. As his condition deteriorated, and he had to use a respirator, his family became alarmed and contacted me, asking to have him admitted to our pulmonary Medical Special Care Unit. It was no easy task, as the unit was fully occupied. I tried to contact our Falk IC, Ames ICU, and Rose CCU – but all were either occupied or had sections unused because of repairs. Finally, one doctor resolved the problem by enabling our gentleman to have a bed in the MSCU. The family was immensely grateful and, accompanied by a physician, brought the patient by night on a chartered plane from New Hampshire. They had insisted on having the patient treated in our hospital and only regained peace of mind when he was settled in our pulmonary unit.

The next afternoon, a Friday, and some time before the Sabbath set in, a physician of that unit contacted me with the patient's request that I lend him phylacteries (tefillin) for prayer. I obliged and helped him in his devotions. How surprised was I when, having finished his prayers with the regular tefillin, and unable to speak because of the tubes in his mouth, he wrote on a pad that he would like me also to get him tefillin arranged according to Rabbenu Tam, which only very pious people use (the regular ones are tefillin by Rashi). In his time of need, this patient's mind continued to be concerned about the fullest possible religious practice. When I visited him again on Saturday, he cried about his inability to worship in a synagogue. I softly murmured a Talmudic statement to him, one discouraging crying on the Sabbath, so he calmed down and pressed my hand into his while I offered him words of comfort and faith.

Persuading Patient to Stay

When I saw her in our psychiatry ward, she insisted on checking herself out. The reason she gave was that her boyfriend would not wait for her. Yet she had been to a few hospitals before coming to us. I dissuaded her from her plan. I pointed out that, once and for all, she must get herself cured and stop hopping from one hospital to the next. Also, she would not be able to maintain her friendship with her boyfriend if she were constantly sick. My recommendation was, therefore, to stay, get treatment, and leave only when her physician judged her to be ready to leave. Meanwhile, her mother too called me to ask for my intervention. I am glad to state that, following our conversation on her floor and after our Sabbath religious services which she attended (and was particularly grateful when I offered a prayer for her recovery at the opened Ark), she stayed on for some two months. As time passed, she gradually came to realize that her condition had improved. At one point, she asked me for a prayer book to take to her room. I obliged by giving her one as a gift. At the end of her stay, she expressed the wish of continuing to come to our Sabbath services after her discharge, since she was going to live in the vicinity of our hospital. I gladly gave her permission to attend, and so, with improved health, and friendship and understanding on our part, she readjusted to regular life on the outside.

Interdating – Conflict Between Young Patient and His Parents

I had seen and spoken to this patient during my regular visits. However, it was at the conclusion of a Saturday morning service that he had particularly enjoyed that he asked for personal guidance. He had a conflict with his parents about interdating. They opposed it, and he felt he had many friends outside the Jewish group and wanted to keep up the relationships. As we all know, this problem of interdating is high on the agenda of the American Jewish community, since it leads to intermarriage, perceived as a danger to our survival as Jews.

I analyzed the problem for him, both from the personal angle and the general Jewish survival angle. I recommended that he share his interest with non-Jewish girls in various clubs of his college, where students meet in groups, but that he should not turn friendly relationships into dating, which usually leads to emotional involvement, and the subsequent problems and conflicts about marriage. He listened carefully, and we parted with the idea that he would give further thought to our conversation.

Russian Jew Comes Closer to Judaism

He was a thirty-two-year-old employee of our hospital, and my family and I had befriended him and invited him to a Rosh Hashanah dinner in our home, where he complained that he had never had the opportunity of being circumcised nor, of course, of celebrating his Bar-Mitzvah. Hearing this, I made the proper contact and had him circumcised by a rabbi, a mohel, who has specialized also in circumcising adults in the presence of a urologist under local anesthesia and for no fee whatsoever. At my request, a urologist at our hospital later checked the circumcision and found it just fine.

Another problem came up. Upon inquiry, this same Russian Jew told me that he was going to work both on Friday night and Saturday afternoon – Yom Kippur – as he feared losing his job. Here again I advised him to trade days with a friendly non-Jewish employee and not to work on the Day of Atonement under any circumstance. This country respects religion, I emphasized to him. He listened to me and was successful in making the switch. He had attended our services on Rosh Hashanah and felt one of my sermons was written especially for him. For Yom Kippur, a neurologist at our hospital had him as his guest in a neighboring synagogue for the full day, which our Russian friend spent in fasting and in prayer.

Now, he still needed to become a Bar-Mitzvah.

The event took place at our hospital's Shemini Atzereth service, on October 18. It so happened that I had the Hebrew text of the blessings in Russian transliteration. He was a Kohen, member of the ancient Hebrew priestly class, and consequently he was called up to the Torah (aliyah) first. He had bought a new tallith (prayer shawl) for the occasion. He did well and was greatly moved by the ceremonial, after which I offered blessings for him and his parents in Russia. That was a very emotional moment for him. At the same time, he derived much pride in his finally having been confirmed and shared the news with all his friends and acquaintances. Now he feels completely comfortable in his full status as a Jew.

Rabbi's Many Ways in Helping

This is another example of the many things a concerned chaplain can do, though such activities are not usually regarded as a chaplain's function.

They had retired to Israel. Then he came to us for delicate surgery for replacement of a heart valve (AVR). His wife came along with him and had me paged as soon as her husband was assigned a bed. She was the worrying type, but there were real problems to handle:

- Blue Cross/Blue Shield: She had continued an American insurance policy but her physician's office had not informed Blue Cross of the need for surgery and the time of stay at our hospital. She was afraid of not being financially covered for the surgery. Therefore, I invited her to my office, and after a couple of calls, I traced the out-of-state branch of Blue Cross in charge and explained the case. I then called the Mount Sinai physician's office and gave them the Blue Cross branch number to notify them officially of the case.
- She needed a place to spend nights during the surgery. I located a neighboring home where she could stay over three nights.
- She needed kosher food. I contacted the Satmar Bikur Cholim ladies, who graciously provided it.

- In the waiting room near our CCU, she was anxious to know how her husband's operation was coming along. I called the OR (operating room) nurse and received a progress report, which gave her assurance.
- For the Sabbath she insisted on staying near her husband's CCU. I obtained permission for the transformation of a doctor's waiting room on the floor into a bedroom for her, through the kind help of the administrator, Cardiac Floor. I had Building Services bring in a cot for her, as well as a refrigerator, and I provided an electric candelabrum for the Sabbath.
- I made regular visits with the patient and arrangements for the wife to stay in a Bikur Cholim apartment the next Sabbath.
- Intervention for discharge on Sunday and not on the Jewish Sabbath.

Finally, after a beautiful recovery, the couple left with happy and grateful feelings.

Conflict Between Supervisor and Patient

This young student had been discharged the day following minor surgery, and the surgeon had noted that in the chart. Still, the patient felt he ought to stay in his room till evening, as he could not move without some pain. It so happened that our Emergency Department insisted on moving a very ill man in his seventies to that floor and the only available bed was that young man's. But he declined to leave. This led the clinical supervisor of H5, to beep me for an immediate visit. I then had a group meeting in the room, which included the supervisor and the young man's parents, who had arrived. There were three options, I explained: to have the young man either stay on a different floor for the day and have him pay for another day of hospitalization, as his physician had already discharged him, or stay in the TV lounge on a couch till the evening, or, of course, go home as the physician recommended. After much deliberation, the parents decided to take him home. Staff helped him into a wheelchair, and the family took him home by taxi.

Determined Refusal

An additional demonstration of the efficacy of the previously mentioned approach occurred in the following case:

My help was requested by a psychiatrist and a male nurse with a young Hassid who could not be induced to take his medicine, eat his meals, drink some fluids, or take a shower – quite an order! First, I obtained a container of orange juice. To gain the full confidence of the patient, I had to get him to trust that what I offered him was religiously permissible. As he sat motionless in the lounge, I approached him, introduced myself, and after telling him he needed fluids to avoid dehydration, I poured him a cup of the juice and asked him to repeat the Hebrew blessing for juice which, of course, he knew well. He listened to me and thirstily drank a few cups of juice, but then the nurse came over and solicited my assistance in having him take his pills. When I presented the pills to him, lo and behold, he easily obliged. Then, explaining to him that words of holiness – i.e. prayer – can only be said with a clean body, I succeeded in having him take a shower as well, something he had refused for some time. Following that, I had a full kosher supper brought to him. In a matter-of-fact manner, I told the patient that religious law required him to wash his hands before eating bread. I led him to the sink, poured water on his hands, made the proper blessing with him and had him sit at the table and eat his meal and helped him physically by cutting his meat with a plastic knife. With just some encouragement, he finished the complete meal, to the surprise of our staff. I then recited the Grace After Meals with him, in Hebrew. I returned to help this patient a number of times, at the repeated requests of his psychiatrist and male nurse.

I elaborate on this case because I want to stress the following point: With this patient, as with the previous one, my approach was to aim my efforts not directly toward eating, taking medicine, or a shower, but toward religious requirements, which I led him to perform. Then, as a result, he did what the hospital staff wanted him to do. Being fully religious, he could not say "no" to religious demands.

Here are clear cases of how understanding the psychology of a Hassid enabled me to make him function better and promote his recovery. I apply the proper individualized approach to each patient, whether religious or not formally observant. I try to understand his thinking and his values, and act accordingly, to the satisfaction of the patient and of the physician's goals. I empathize with the patient and help lead him on the road to recovery as prescribed by his physician.

It is my empirical conclusion that it would be of considerable help, particularly in psychiatry, to have some religious staff who could better relate to religious patients because of their own knowledge of Jewish observance.

Miraculous Recovery

He was a pious Israeli who had been a patient at our hospital for some three months, two of which were spent in our Cardiac CU with complications of renal failure and infection. He was given sedatives so that he would not disconnect the tubes attached to him, and thus slept through the entire Jewish High Holy Day season. It is due in great measure to the uninterrupted and dedicated efforts of our nursing staff that, against all odds, he made a marvelous recovery. During that time, I was in constant touch with his wife and two sons, arranged their sleeping over on the eve of the Jewish Sabbath and holidays in a waiting room near the cardiac unit, and offered counsel and comfort. Due to the language difficulty, I regularly helped them talk to the doctors and nurses. When the patient could finally converse, I told him that verse 4 of Psalm 136 truly applied to him. It reads: "[O give thanks] to Him Who alone does great marvels: for His loving-kindness lasts forever."

Only After Uttering a Blessing

When I approached this psychiatric patient – a physician – his wife told me that he does not talk. Still, holding my ethrog and lulav during Sukkoth, I invited him to repeat after me the two required blessings: one thanking God for the harvest season and the second for the gift of life. To everybody's surprise, he recited both blessings in Hebrew while wearing a skullcap I had placed on his head and holding the religious symbols in his hands. He knew me from previous visits, and, I guess, wanted to be nice to a rabbi!

Hassidic Couple's Conflict

The associate director of Nursing Affairs asked for my intervention in this case, in which the clinical supervisor and the social worker were involved. It concerned a seriously ill child in Falk Pediatrics whose Hassidic parents were separated. The father, who had not seen his family for more than a year, suddenly appeared in the hospital, to the consternation of his wife, who had him evicted by Security. Yet the father came back. At my suggestion and in my presence, he saw the child who was amiable to him, thus proving that the wife's fears of adverse effects were without foundation. The Hassidic Rabbinic Court, which, so the wife claimed, had forbidden him to visit the child, called to deny that, adding that they do not issue such written rulings. The physician of the child also clearly told this quarreling couple that, according to our rules, both parents are equally entitled to see the child all day. He urged them to resolve their conflict as mature adults, which, unfortunately, they could not do. Therefore, I worked out a schedule of separate visits, allowing specific times to husband and wife. I had both of them sign that agreement, which was handed over to the social workers, with the understanding that if any of the two violated the agreement, Security would be called in to enforce it. This put an end to the fighting. The agreement worked.

"It's in Your Favor"

He was a patient in our new Cardiac Intensive Care Unit called 5E CCU. There were no empty beds available in one of the regular units, so he was kept in the CCU. He felt better and resented the fact that he was not moved.

He would have gone to a private room, he said, but would have had to pay an extra sum, which his insurance company would not cover, so he was grouchy and angry. My way of handling him was to point out two advantages in his present setup. First of all, he received an extra day or days of full supervision and monitoring – and that is always a plus. Then, he had a beautiful, private enclosure in our new building for no extra charge. Those two points in his favor impressed him, and all he could say was that he was grateful for my enlightening him. "Now, please relax," I told him as he shook my hand.

"You Put a New Soul into Me"

He was undergoing chemotherapy and had requested to talk to me privately. He then related to me the history of his illness and its treatment, saying that he was worried about the future. We chatted for a long while. As I recited a Hebrew prayer for his recovery and wished him well, he lifted up his head from his pillow, shook my hand warmly, and thanking me for my visit, added, "You put a new soul into me."

Hungry on Passover

On an intermediate day of Passover, a call for help came on my voice mail. It turned out that this young mother had been told by the physician to stay for a number of hours in our Emergency Unit in order to observe her infant, whose diagnosis was difficult to establish. In addition, she had brought along an older child. They had not eaten since breakfast, and long hours of waiting still awaited them. They were all hungry and urgently needed kosher food for Passover. I turned both to our catering department and to our kitchen and obtained a box of matzahs, a bottle of Kedem grape juice, and two packs of gefilte fish and, like Abraham of the Bible, brought them over to our distressed guests

Count Your Blessings

In Gynecology, I found a young woman in tears while her husband was standing at her bedside all bewildered. The surgeon had told her that chances are that she may not have a second child. Upon inquiry, it turned out that the removed tissue proved to be benign. I, therefore, called her attention to the importance of that fact, which means that her health was good, and she would live and be able to raise her four-year-old son. Concerning a second child, the future would determine its advisability. In the meantime, she ought to count her blessings and be grateful for her own health and the loving family that she had. Her crying subsided as she became aware of the good side of her situation.

Our Admiration for the Neurosurgeon and His Anesthesiologist

Beginning on the Seder night when this young Israeli nursing teacher was brought to the hospital's Seder hall with her mother, I had established a personal rapport with both. I visited them frequently and often prayed for her. On the day of surgery for a tumor in the spinal column, I sat with the mother through an evening of waiting for the surgeon and listening to his report following surgery. It was an agonizing experience, as the prognosis proved ominous. The grief-stricken mother was in need of a great deal of emotional and spiritual support. I wish to express my deep admiration for the neurosurgeon, who worked hard and long on the operation and then spent a long time explaining the situation to the mother with great patience, understanding, and deep sympathy. Recognizing that the patient's coming to this country and stay at the hospital was paid by monetary gifts from nurses and doctors throughout Israel, and the balance by Bikur Cholim, the neurosurgeon waived his fee and so did the anesthesiologist. I also wish to praise our Social Work Department for their exceptionally selfless efforts and assistance in every way. Mother and daughter have since returned to Israel.

Must It Be an Ivy League School?

This young man had been a scholarship student in one of our Ivy League colleges and in an outstanding English university, where his health failed him and made him just pass. Upon his return to this country, five prominent law schools turned down his application. He got into a depression. He was also alienated from his parents and was living by himself. He felt hopeless and helpless. I offered him two guiding points: (1) Not to sign himself out of our hospital, as he was about to do, but wait till the psychiatrist discharged him; and (2) to apply to non-Ivy League law schools and develop excellence in one branch of law and a good rapport with one professor. That will help him practice a profession he likes, earn a livelihood, and receive recognition for the mastery of his specialty. Above all, there was no need to let his rejection from prominent law schools affect his health, his self-image, and his future. There is more than one road to happiness and success. He was persuaded and stayed till his official discharge and also promised to consider my second recommendation seriously.

7: SOME PERSONAL CONVERSION PROBLEMS

Adoptive Jewish Parents

This was a very unusual case. Her adoptive Jewish parents were opposed to religion and had not converted her when she was young. Now an adult, a staff member of our hospital, and academically highly educated, she had studied Judaism, fell in love with it, and began practicing most of its requirements. She wanted to be officially converted by an Orthodox rabbi. "Even my genes are religious," she added. It appeared to me that she was completely sincere. To her, Judaism was like air to breathe. There was no ulterior motive whatever. Whereupon, I called up a former classmate of mine who handles conversions, and referred her to him. That young lady and former doctoral academician wrote to me: "I am so glad I spoke to you, and I can't wait until everything is official and done." She was converted in time for Rosh Hashanah.

Conversion? Rather Remain in Her Own Religion

She served as a secretary to a member of our administration. She had read up on Judaism on her own and requested an appointment with me. She told me that a book which particularly impressed her was entitled *The Rabbinic Mind*, written by a Jewish scholar. Her religion was Baptist. What she wanted was to discuss possible conversion to Judaism. In our conversation, I pointed out to her the two major problems:

- She was proposing to join a people that has suffered and been persecuted throughout the centuries. Being black, her history too was replete with suffering, discrimination, and persecution. So why have a double dose of it?
- Difficulties in practicing the Jewish religion in an environment in which we are a minority and in which the majority follows a different calendar and different festivals and mores, etc. A non-Jew does not have to refrain from work on Saturday, the Jewish Sabbath, and on Jewish holidays. He/she may eat any food. However, being Jewish, eating

nonkosher foods and working on Sabbath and Holidays are transgressions.

She was an intelligent young lady. At that time, she was about to return to her native South. I advised her not to rush things, but rather take time to reflect deeply. I also stressed that, according to the Jewish religion, non-Jews attain paradise by practicing just the seven basic universal laws for humanity, called the Laws of Noah, while a Jew must observe the great number of laws of the Torah to attain the same goal. My advice to her was to remain within her own religion but to be a friend of the Jewish people.

A few years later, I received a letter from her thanking me for my explanations and stating that she did decide to remain in her own religion and would, indeed, always be a friend of the Jewish people.

August 22, 1994
Rabbi Charles Spirn
The Mount Sinai Medical Center
Fifth Avenue & 100th Street
New York, N.Y. 10029

Dear Good Samaritan,

I just wanted to take the time to thank you again for advice you gave me in 1982 or 1983 when I worked as a temporary secretary at Mount Sinai.

I was merely passing through but you took the time to answer my questions or to provoke me to answer them myself by not answering them.

You are a very dear person. You will not be forgotten – not ever.

May God bless you more and more each day.

Non-Jewish Top Administrator Describes His Relationship with the Jewish Chaplain

May 15, 1992

Dear Rabbi Spirn:

I want to say with great sincerity that I will miss you when I leave Mount Sinai. You have always been caring and considerate to me, both professionally and personally. I will not forget that you have gone out of your way for me on more than one occasion.

I appreciate your participation in my party. Thank you for contributing to the gift. You can continue to support me with your prayers. You will be pleased to know that I have again become an active believer in God and an active member of my church.

I wish you and your family all good fortune.

Sincerely,
Dr. ---

From a New Returnee to Judaism

Dear Rabbi:

May you and your family be inscribed for a good year, Elul 29, 5752, September 27, 1992. You were a great moral booster to me all the many times you visited me when I was in reverse isolation, bringing me *The Jewish Press* and bottles of grape juice. Later, when I was able to attend the Shabbat services, I was moved almost to tears at times to remember that God's presence is always with us, even in the hospital. And perhaps especially in the hospital. My catheter was removed – chemotherapy is a thing of the past, *Baruch Hashem* (Blessed be God) – and my blood levels are nearing normal.

I have been back to working steady at the Metropolitan Museum of Art for the past four weeks, even working overtime the past four Saturday nights (Sundays) from which I am writing you this card. You do a great service for the Jewish sick in this world, and may God reward you in this world and the world to come. You deserve it, if anyone does. I am using a sick day and Labor Day to observe Rosh Hashanah at the Kehilath Jeshurun Beginners' Service – a service for Jews who are returning and some who never even had a chance to learn (like the Soviet Jews). Perhaps when more of my energy returns, I will come to visit the sick and see you, but not in my pajamas or hospital gown. Thank you for your prayers.

Sincerely,

Begins Talking at Torah

He attended our Sabbath morning services where, since we had a minyan (quorum), I read the Torah. I called up every male present. I also called up this patient, encouraged him to come forward and assisted him in making the blessings at the Torah. After the service, a nurse from Psychiatry revealed to me that this patient was on her floor and had refused to talk, so that his saying the blessings aloud were the first words he had uttered for some time. With this precedent, she hoped he would open up and start communicating with others too.

"God Needs You Too"

She had undergone open heart surgery and her husband, wearing a skullcap, talked to her at her bedside in CCU, trying to cheer her up. She looked comfortable but a bit worried. After having offered a prayer at her bedside, I added: "You need God, sure enough. But remember, God needs you too, you who are on His team." These last words brought hope and cheer to both the patient and her husband.

"Handle with Care"

She had an English last name from which it was impossible to guess that she was Jewish, and her name was not on the list of Jewish patients. Her mother stopped me in the hall and asked for my visit. It turned out that this mother had already solicited the visit of an outside rabbi for the express purpose of making her daughter more religious. She also prayed aloud in her daughter's room and kept on arguing with the daughter about the practice of religion. I sat in the room, trying to assess the situation.

The daughter, who had intermarried and was now divorced, revealed that she had undergone very serious surgery at our hospital; the surgeon had told her later that she almost died on the operating table when something unexpected occurred that saved her life. Our patient ascribed this to Divine intervention and proclaimed her strong belief in the existence of God. Her mother, however, who had not given that daughter any religious education – due to poverty, she claimed – was now uninterruptedly pushing her daughter to religious practice, which the daughter rejected.

I had a very difficult time to get this overbearing mother to desist from her preaching to a middle-aged daughter. She promised to leave her daughter in peace only when I cautioned her privately that her action might trigger off a worse problem, necessitating a transfer to Psychiatry. I told her this situation was fragile. "Handle it with care." This finally registered with the mother. As for the daughter, I answered some of her questions and her request for books on Judaism and sided with her against her mother's approach. I calmed her, stressed the need for peace of mind during her convalescence, and the need for emotional support, leaving the question of religious practice to the future development. She was most appreciative of my concern and attitude.

Interdating

A young patient, a college student, daughter of divorced parents, went to live with her father, a Hassid, after the death of her mother. At school, she had begun interdating. When her father found out about it, he strongly objected, and she too realized it was not in her best interest to continue that relationship. Now, she wanted to shift to a Jewish-sponsored college. I briefed her on such schools.

Dates of Permitted Marriages

A resident physician stopped me to inquire about the summer period of three weeks, during which Jewish weddings may not be solemnized since these are periods of mourning for the Jewish people. I gave her the information, encouraged her to select a happy date, and handed over to her a card with blessing of the Sabbath lights, which she promised to use.

"You Gave Me Courage"

When the going was rough and medical prognosis on the pessimistic side, I helped a lady patient keep up hope which, with time, proved justified. She said to me: "You gave me courage by stressing to me that the final word has not been spoken yet in my case, and that ultimately God will have the last word. Thank you, Rabbi. Indeed, God has been good to me."

Conversion? Not Needed

He came to my office all excited. He wanted to be converted to Judaism because he loved the Jewish religion while his parents were atheists. I had him relax first. Then realizing that he was a medical student at our School of Medicine and that he was of Jewish background, I asked him whether his parents were Jewish. Yes, he answered, they were both Jewish but atheists, and he wanted none of that. "I want to be a full Jew" – he insisted. How astonished was he when I told him that he was a Jew by birth and needed no conversion. "Is there anything I need to do to be a full Jew?" he persisted. It turned out that he was not circumcised. Whereupon, I recommended that he undergo circumcision and made a referral for him to a Jewish organization that provides proper circumcision to adults. Now he felt at ease with himself. A few weeks later, he returned to me to tell me that he was circumcised and glad to have it done. He added: "I am going to take a leave of absence from the Medical School, go to a yeshiva in Rockland County to study the Jewish faith and live as a full Jew."

Counseling Staff – Jewish and Non-Jewish

I am glad to have enjoyed the trust and confidence of our numerous staff. Members of our Medical Center's various departments, including physicians, have been guided by me in their personal as well as religious problems. They have had their problems clarified and possible solutions offered or referrals made. Though my identity as a rabbi is clearly known, some non-Jewish staff members have also requested meetings with me with reference to their personal problems. These cases remain private and confidential. My reward is that I have helped people in their dilemmas or conflicts and added a measure of relief as well as of peace of mind and peace of soul.

8: SUFFERING AND FEAR

Advice to Divorcee

At Sabbath morning services which she attended, she related that she was civilly divorced and that she was waiting for her former husband to come to New York from the West Coast, where he now resided, to go through the procedures for a Jewish divorce (called a *get*). I brought her a sense of relief when I advised her that the wait was not necessary: her former husband can go to a rabbinic court in his West Coast city, arrange the *get*, and then the court will, through its rabbinic messengers, deliver the divorce to her in New York. Both parties need not be present simultaneously according to Jewish law.

Learns About Amicable Settlement of Differences

She attended our Sabbath services. A sermon I delivered, about the functions of a Jewish judge according to the Torah, struck home with her. Disputes had arisen between her and her former husband in the course of their divorce proceedings. And so what particularly appealed to her in my sermon was the Jewish concept that a judge ought to look for compromise and mutual agreement between the litigating parties, so that both remain friends and not become enemies after the trial. She longed for that approach, which does not concentrate on the case alone and making one a victor and the other a loser who will hate his opponent, but rather put stress on resolving the problem amicably, so that a good human rapport remains among the litigants toward each other.

Upon her request, I sent her a copy of the sermon which, most probably, she will forward to her former husband with the idea that he too come to terms of divorce with her in an amicable way.

"Draw on Your Friends"

She became troubled as she was told that she would have to return to our hospital for treatment. She particularly bemoaned the fact that she was needed at home to take care of a sick husband and a sick son. My advice to her was that this was the time to draw on family and friends to extend a helping hand. The popular saying that a friend in need is a friend indeed should be tested now among those whom she considered friends. The patient promised to follow this advice and felt more relaxed.

Quadruple Heart Bypass

A colleague of mine gave her my telephone number, and she called in anticipation of her husband's checking into our hospital. On the day of surgery, I was in constant touch with her and met her toward the evening in Annenberg 8. As her husband had made her promise not to see him on the day of surgery, I became her link with our CCU, where he was recuperating after quadruple heart bypass surgery. The nurse in charge graciously offered to call her up late at night to tell her about her husband's condition. The wife requested that I call her the next morning, since I have access to the CCU. This case, as so many others, just highlights the trust people have in clergy, in or out of a hospital.

A Young Judge's Crisis

He had been deaf in one ear since childhood and now suffered acoustic neurinoma (a nerve tumor) in the other ear. He had come to our hospital from the Midwest for surgery by one of our top specialists. On the day before surgery, he became very anxious and frightened and asked for the rabbi's prompt visit. He talked about his life and his fear of total hearing loss. I succeeded in making him regain a measure of calm and hope, and promised to see him after surgery. Unfortunately, the operation did not save his hearing. His wife had briefed me that he had talked of suicide if he were to lose his hearing. To my written question to him on how he felt, he responded with thumb down. I wrote some comforting words and returned to him again and again. He had managed to decipher lip reading and I made him count his blessings, reassured him about his livelihood as he had just been elected judge: since he was an appellate judge whose decisions mostly involved reading the case and writing his decision, he could well continue in his job. His wife had done much research on new machines that could be of help to him, and much sooner than I expected, he left our hospital in good spirits.

Needed Her Daughter

I found this patient upset because her daughter, a Manhattan resident, refused to visit her, claiming that her mother did not need hospitalization – so the mother said. I contacted her daughter personally, and she visited her mother as a result of my call.

Bone Marrow Transplants

She was all of twelve and spent long periods of time at our hospital, suffering from leukemia. When her situation worsened, a brother of hers, who had been studying at a yeshiva in Israel, returned to give her a bone marrow transplant. I also witnessed two additional similar cases at our hospital: one of a sister giving it to a brother and, the other, of a sister-in-law giving it to a brother-in-law. Jewish family bonds are indeed powerful, regardless of the degree of formal religious observances.

The Road Not to Be Taken

She had had cancer surgery, and though the surgeon had done a thorough job, she was very upset and afraid of the future. "Now," I told her, "two roads are open before you. One is to worry, be tearful, and make yourself and your family miserable – and with all that accomplish nothing. The alternative is to do what the Jewish religion recommends: thank God for every new day, be confident in God's mercy, live one day at a time fully and positively, be grateful for it and for the beautiful family with which you are blessed, and do good deeds. The sage Hillel used to say, 'Blessed be the Lord every single day.' Imitate Hillel and may God watch over you and bestow long life on you." The patient listened attentively, relaxed, wiped off her tears, and looked reassured and hopeful.

"Give Us Some Words of Comfort, of Wisdom"

I had seen that patient very often during his wait for a liver transplant. When some problems developed after the transplant, which, however, his physician had identified and was treating, his wife asked me for something positive, something comforting and wise that would help them gain peace of mind. My reply: the first half of good news is that the physician has identified the problem – it is much more worrisome when the diagnosis has not been established and a search for it continues. The second half is that it is treatable. Both those factors should give the patient and his wife a great measure of peace of mind. I left this couple in much better spirits.

Patient Describes Chaplain's Unique Role in His Recovery

March 3, 1997

Dear Director:

I have been a patient at the Mount Sinai Hospital since November 12, 1996. I received a new heart on February 21, 1997. By the grace of God, the new heart came just in time.

Mount Sinai Hospital has a staff of physicians and nurses who gave me a confidence I never thought would be possible for an operation of this kind. They treated this miracle as an everyday occurrence. In the time I have been here, *all* these operations were successful.

More important than all the doctors and nurses was the attention and loving care from Rabbi Charles Spirn. He is a "mensch." I'm proud to know that this man represents the Jewish faith to the outside world because he is kind, caring, and humble. Whenever he visited me, he lifted my spirits and did everything possible for my well-being.

I am proud to tell you my feelings in this letter.

Sincerely,

Unworthy of Being a Martyr?

She was tearful and adjusted poorly to being hospitalized. I let her vent her feelings. After revealing that she had been in the Auschwitz extermination camp where her family perished in the Holocaust, in her distress she suddenly added that she wished she had perished there, too, but God had not found her worthy of becoming a martyr. It took great empathy and patience to redirect her thoughts to the view that she had remained alive for a purpose, and she should sanctify God's name in life. I left her in better control of her emotions. A week later she was discharged, presumably in improved health.

Martyrdom is the highest expression of religion; it means giving one's life to God. However, one can also be a martyr by doing extraordinary deeds for God in life. I directed this patient toward that second form of martyrdom.

"Rabbi Handled Issues for Us Even Before We Thought Of Them"

Dear Director:

We wish to advise you of the constructive, sensitive role of Rabbi Charles A. Spirn. My wife's illness and her surgery came upon us quite suddenly. Our degree of dislocation, upset and confusion was severe, despite the doctor's precise, wonderful care. We are observant Orthodox Jews. Paramedical issues that a physician simply cannot address – no matter how skillful and thoughtful – presented themselves to us. Rabbi Spirn handled them all smoothly. He handled issues for us even before we thought of them. He answered questions wisely. He gave excellent advice, freely (he was always accessible, to advise, or to do some important favor). He was active, intervening in issues of room selection, and other key issues. Nothing is too much for Rabbi Spirn. His home is warm and open. He is there – and how much we needed him to be there! We compliment you on him and thank you for your superior hospital and personnel.

Respectfully,

Priority to Parent or to Daughter?

Our Patient Representative Department referred this case to me. Her father was in a coma at one of our ICUs, and her mother had been spending her days at his bedside. She too had come from out-of-town to offer emotional support, especially to her mother. A divorcee, she had brought along her teenage daughter, who had threatened to commit suicide. Now she was faced with a dilemma: return home with her daughter, who had been accepted for psychological therapy, or stay here near her parents. Upon inquiry, it turned out that, though this out-of-town family had neither relatives nor friends in our metropolitan area who would pitch in with hospital visits, there was yet a married brother to whose home the mother returned at night. That fact led me to suggest a solution to this guilt-ridden lady.

I explained it to her in the following way: There is little physical or emotional help she could give to a comatose father. Our physicians are doing their utmost for him, she agreed, and all she could do is add her prayers for his recovery. Concerning her mother, I find it of great value that, after spending a day at the hospital, she retreats at night to the warm atmosphere of her son's home, where she can share her concerns and find a measure of understanding, affection, and relief. Moreover, because the brother is a New Yorker, he may find some friend who will spend a couple of hours some days with his mother at the hospital in addition to his own visits. All that adds up to giving priority to the needs of the teenage daughter, whom no one except she can take care of. I also alerted her to taking seriously a teenager's talking about suicide. It is a cry for help – prompt help. Therefore, I advised her to return home and get her daughter into treatment. She had requested to speak to a rabbi to unburden herself and, most surely, to guide her in her dilemma.

The Starved Professor – "Rabbi, Please Get Me Some Food"

As I made regular rounds, this patient asked me to do him "a big favor" and get him something to eat or to drink. He said he was literally starving after a few days of testing. My reaction was to check with the nurse who, in my presence, looked up this patient's chart, which stated that beginning at 2:00 P.M. that day, he was allowed fluids by mouth. Since it was already 3:00 P.M., I urged the nurse not to have him wait for supper but to give him something in the meantime. She brought him jello. The patient was overwhelmingly grateful to me. It turned out that he was a professor of philosophy at a big metropolitan college. He said that he now discovered that his reliance on Spinoza and stoicism was not helpful and that he preferred my Jewish ethics. He also told me that he decided to observe Yom Kippur, which he had not done before.

Message from the Lubavitcher Rebbe

The wife of a prominent Israeli rabbi called me. She had consulted the Lubavitcher Rebbe (Hassidic sage) in Brooklyn who, upon hearing that her husband was a patient at the Mount Sinai Hospital, told her to deliver to me, its Jewish chaplain, the message that I should give her husband "very special attention." I felt very honored by this great sage's confidence in me. I did check with the nursing staff and found out that the patient's cancer had not affected any vital organ. However, he was depressed and refused to eat and to walk. He was a very intelligent man and had full understanding of his illness – which worked to his detriment. I was able to get him to walk and drink and raise his spirits. I saw him twice daily till he returned to Israel.

A Jewish Pope?

As I made my rounds in the Intensive Care Unit where the Lubavitcher Rebbe was a patient, the floor's nurses stopped me to ask, "Is he the Jewish Pope?"

My answer: "No. We have no Pope in the Jewish religion. However, he is a towering spiritual personality, among the greatest in this century."

I was most grateful to our hospital for the long weeks of care given to the Lubavitcher Rebbe, and the utmost respect with which they treated him and his hundreds of disciples who crowded around the hospital praying for his recovery.

Fear of Violating the Sabbath

Her rabbi recommended that she contact me. Her husband, an outpatient, was scheduled for a Friday midafternoon liver biopsy, after which he was to remain in the Recovery Room and then be discharged. Problem: fear of not being able to return home before the Sabbath begins. Solution: I called up the physician, explained the couple's predicament, and suggested that the biopsy be forwarded to Friday morning. The physician obliged as a special favor to a Sabbath-observing family.

Volume on Talmud Photocopied

A social worker called me about seeing a young Iranian-Jewish outpatient, very poor, and assisting him in resolving a problem. He had borrowed a

Persian exposition on the Talmud, its methodology and content, and wanted it photocopied for personal study. The social worker and I worked together on this project, xeroxing page after page on the hospital's copier, since the patient was too poor to have it done professionally.

Visiting and Praying with the Klausenberger Rebbe

One more outstanding Hassidic sage, the Klausenberger Rebbe, was a patient at our hospital, and I made regular visits to him. I introduced myself as an Orthodox rabbi. After some talk about Judaism, he gave me a blessing that I should always find grace in the sight of people I meet. Later, as he held my hand in his, I wished him a speedy recovery and to continue being a spiritual shepherd in the Jewish community.

I also had the privilege of joining him at special Friday evening services, which were held in the Conference Room of G-6. The minyan (quorum of ten males) was guaranteed by the presence of some of his young disciples, who spent the Sabbath with him at our hospital. This afforded me a special occasion to pray together with this charismatic personality and to observe the great respect and love given to him by his disciples.

I particularly wish to thank our hospital for allowing this number of visitors in the Conference Room. In turn, the Hassidim subdued their voices during prayer so as not to inconvenience or disturb patients and staff on the floor. Their spending the Sabbath on our premises evoked respect to them and credit to their rebbe.

"No Visitors Please" – but Rabbi Is Welcome

From time to time, one comes across a sign on a patient's door reading, "No visitors please." In general, the only thing to do is to leave my card at the door, and I usually do so. However, I have also experimented with knocking on the door, announcing my name and asking, "May I come in?" The answer I mostly receive is, "Please come in," and we have a friendly chat. When I return a week later, the patient usually remembers my name and is glad to see me. For such patients, the rabbi is not just "a visitor" but a source of unique help and uplift.

4:30 A.M. Reveille on the Sabbath

Early Saturday, we were awakened at 4:30 A.M. by the uninterrupted ringing of our home phone. In religious law, one is not allowed to pick up the receiver on the Sabbath, so we couldn't respond, but were very worried. Who could possibly persist in calling for forty-five minutes? Only then did our doorbell ring. Two of the hospital's security men came to inform a young rabbi, our guest for the Sabbath (because his wife had given birth on Friday), that he was urgently needed at the hospital. After he had rushed out as quickly as he could, I felt I should go as well and be available in case of need.

It turned out that his wife had become panicky when her newborn son developed a breathing problem and had to be taken to the Infant ICU in KP9. I promptly joined the father at the ICU. We were relieved after some time, when the physician in charge reported to us that the condition of the child had improved, but he would still remain in the unit for a few days of observation. Dressed in hospital gowns, we approached the one-day-old infant, and I offered for him the prayer for the recovery of the sick. We then conveyed the good news to the mother and urged her, at the recommendation of the doctor, to visit the child herself, and regain her peace of mind after this big scare.

I am glad to state that the child improved as expected and went home with his mother for the following Sabbath. I would like to point out here that the only way to reach the chaplain during any emergency on the Sabbath is to send a messenger to his home.

Unload for Health's Sake!

She carried three jobs, each one taxing by itself. This overload landed her in our hospital. We had a friendly chat, and she showed me a booklet of Hebrew prayers that she was using in her daily worship. It surprised me to see a young, single woman in her twenties burdening herself beyond endurance. I encouraged her to make an agenda, place her health on the top of it, as number one, and guide herself accordingly. Whatever undermined her health should be discarded, unloaded. She should earn a living without trying to become a Rockefeller financially. I gave her some pamphlets for inspiration, and she promised to take a serious reconsideration of her priorities and needs.

"Sent from Heaven"

I found her in pain and discomfort. As I introduced myself, she immediately responded that she liked my articles published in *The Jewish Press*. Her daughter held her right hand and a physician with a long needle was making taps from the lung for a culture. This took some time, and in order to take her mind off her pain, I held her left hand in mine and questioned her about her family, to which she gladly responded. She had great pride in her pious forebears and in her equally pious children and grandchildren. Relating this occupied her so intensely that the physician could proceed without her crying. When the procedure was completed, she exclaimed, "You were sent from heaven just at the right moment to help me in my distress!"

Da, Da, Oui, Oui

Realizing from this patient's name that she was Russian, which I do not speak, I asked her whether she spoke Yiddish. "*Nyet!*" she answered. How about another language?

"*Parlez-vous français?*" I took a chance in asking her.

"*Da, da – oui, oui,*" she answered. "*Je parle français.*" And so we had an interesting conversation in French. She was so happy to relate to me in a language that we both knew. Indeed, in a hospital of our size and renown, one meets patients from many parts of the world, and it is a mutual pleasure for me and for them to find a way to relate to each other.

Gratefulness of Staff

September 3, 1996

Dear Rabbi Spirn,

You were so extremely helpful in facilitating the difficult and complicated discharge last week. Both the nurse manager and I would like to compliment, commend, and thank you for the comfort you were able to provide the distraught daughter and the confidence you were able to gain. Without your generous participation, a satisfactory solution to the daughter's concerns and an unchallenged discharge would have been very difficult to achieve.

Sincerely yours,

Brain Surgery of a Physician

He was a highly intelligent man. He felt surgery was the best solution to his problem and seemed to accept it. He was very friendly toward me and also attended our Sabbath services. When I offered a prayer for his recovery at the Torah, he had tears in his eyes. Later, following surgery, his condition improved, and he joined us again at services. He always felt cheered by my presence and appreciative of my friendship toward him.

A Patient to His Attorney: "The Rabbi Is Like a Father to Me"

He had come to this country from Iran and had obtained a degree in engineering. Unfortunately, while he was walking on 59th Street, a woman threw herself off a roof, landed on him and died. He had multiple injuries and spent more than three months at our hospital where I saw him, counseled him, and befriended him. Two-and-a-half years after that incident, the case still had not been settled, and he was worried about its outcome, unable as he was to do any work. I offered to speak to his lawyer on the phone and did so with this former patient in my office. When the attorney claimed he could not divulge information to me, I handed over the receiver to our young Iranian Jew who said, "The rabbi is like a father to me. You may speak to him openly." Hopefully, this telephone call will somewhat hasten the progress of the case. It certainly carried an implicit message to the lawyer that his client is not alone, but that a rabbi is watching that no injustice be done to this lonely victim. He continues to attend our Sabbath services, which also give him an occasion to unburden himself about his broken career, his physical pain, and his legal complications, which had been needlessly dragged out.

"When Will I See You Again?"

She was a very lonely, elderly patient. Her link to life was an only child, a son, whom, at her suggestion, I called up, inviting him to visit his mother more frequently. Whenever I saw her, she expressed joy at my taking an interest in her and, at parting, would ask loudly, "When will I see you again?" In return, I gave her a specific date of two days later and always kept my promise. Her action reminded me of the wish of the Jewish Rip Van Winkle, Honi Hamaagel: "Give me company or give me death."

Survivor Finds Rabbi Understands Human Suffering

She was a descendant of a well-known, prominent Hassidic dynasty. Her sufferings in Poland and later transfer to Siberia, where her young parents had died of the cold weather and starvation, plus the recent loss of her husband, had embittered her to the extent that she did not care to live anymore. She had also refrained from having children, she said, because she did not want to bring them into this cruel world. I listened to the story of her bitter life and let her unburden herself. When I told her that I too had experienced suffering in Western Europe during World War II, it established some rapport between us, for she felt that I could understand her well. She declined to ignite the Sabbath lights, and I did not insist. I visited her regularly and tried to inject some cheer into her life. Weeks later, when a roommate of hers she had befriended asked for the Sabbath candelabrum, I suggested sending her one too. This time, she accepted. Her outlook had become a bit more optimistic. Hope for recovery had strengthened her will to live.

Nephew Briefed About Terminal Aunt

I found the nephew at the bedside of this terminally ill patient; he had come from Paris to be near his aunt. He turned to me for explanations of Jewish law on what to do during expiration and how to make preparations for the funeral. We conversed in French since he spoke little English. I briefed him on Jewish tradition in this respect and also gave him mimeographed texts of prayers appropriate for the situation.

Growth on Liver or Kidney?

This elderly patient was advised to have surgery to determine whether a growth was on the liver, in which case it would be inoperable, or on the kidney, and then one kidney could be removed safely. The hesitation proved to be a terrible ordeal for the family till, after consultation with physicians and rabbis knowledgeable in medicine, they resolved the conflict in favor of surgery. Fortunately for this patient, the growth was on the kidney. This patient stayed at our hospital more than five weeks, and I visited him regularly. I also guided the family through the hard time of the patient's confusion when he called home at midnight and claimed there was a fire in the hospital, and he was trying to leave his bed. I established direct phone contact between the wife and the supervising nurse on the floor for use in case of need. My wife and I also welcomed the patient's wife in our home every Sabbath and during a snowstorm. The patient's wife writes: "My warmest thanks for your hospitality. We are remembering your thoughtfulness and warmly thanking you because there is something especially nice in everything you do."

"I Want You to Encourage Me"

She had made a wonderful recovery, and she was grateful to God for it. Now, as she prepared to go home, she asked me for some prayer texts that I had given her during her illness, as she had misplaced them. While obliging, I also offered her the card with the blessings on the Sabbath lights, telling her that I wanted to encourage her to light candles at home every week in honor of the Jewish Sabbath. Her response – most positive – was: "I want you to encourage me to carry out all Jewish traditions."

Mastectomy

An hour before surgery, this mastectomy patient called the office of Patient Representative to request my visit. Fear had gotten the best of her. The very appearance of the rabbi helped her overcome her loneliness at this critical time in her life. We know what is on the mind of such a patient: the risk of surgery: Is it malignant or benign? is it metastatic or localized? disfigurement? facing the future? My visit apparently did her good in preparing her emotionally for the surgery. She said she felt relieved, calmed, and hopeful. I visited her again the next day, a Friday, as I had promised. I found her relaxed and at peace with herself. I suggested she light the Sabbath electric candles we provide, and she gladly accepted. She told me she would introduce this tradition to her home as well. She was discharged soon afterwards and gratefully bid me good-bye.

"Last Rites?" God Needs You Here

She remembered that half a year ago, at our hospital and at the request of her children, I had given her what she called the "last rites" (the Confession – *Viduy* – and the prayer for the dying) as they felt she was terminal. And now, she was still alive and back in our hospital. "What happened?" she asked me. The answer, I told her, is that when we offer those last prayers at the request of family, we stress that it does not mean that the patient's life is sure to end. It does mean that he or she wants to be at peace with God, Who alone makes the ultimate decision. In her case, as we see it, God wanted her and needed her in *this* world, and she should be grateful for that. Hearing that, her face brightened, and she kept repeating, "God still needs me in this world."

Eyesight Problem Patient

This patient, who had eye surgery at our hospital, was unable to pursue normal reading. I put him in contact with In-Touch Network, which distributes special radios for listening to their day-long programs for people who cannot read standard print. I also recommended that he contact the Library for the Blind and the Jewish Braille Institute, with the latter having tapes on Jewish topics. I had become aware of the above when I was interviewed by Dr. Ruth Klebaner of the In-Touch Network, and I passed on the information to help patients.

Obtaining Ten-Hour Pass for Patient

He had been at our hospital for five months in the Inpatient Rehabilitation Department. Having only one leg, he moved around in a wheelchair. He was afraid of incurring financial disaster, since his only permanent employee was soon to retire, and he needed permission to travel by car to Philadelphia to transfer his business to New York. A Bikur Cholim rabbi of the Lubavitcher Hassidic movement of Brooklyn was to drive him, and a young man who had been trained at our hospital to handle a patient in a wheelchair was to accompany them. I was glad to have been instrumental in securing the necessary pass for him to leave for ten hours. As I explained to the physician involved, this was necessary to assure the patient's livelihood after he was discharged from the hospital. The doctors understood the situation and complied with my request, to the satisfaction of our patient.

Courage and Fortitude – "Thanks for Caring"

Dear Dr. Spirn:

I cannot tell you how helpful you were to me with your spiritual guidance at the time of my most trying moments prior and subsequent to my surgery.

Your inspirational attitude gave me the courage and fortitude to face my *second* open heart surgery.

May you continue to carry on your work for many, many years to come.

Thanks for caring.

Happy New Year for you and the ones you love.

A Subway Victim – Helping an Invalid

He had been in an accident: Either he had fallen off the platform of a subway or someone had pushed him off just as a train was arriving. One leg was amputated and a finger of a hand was missing. He was a religious man and requested a prayer book, a Soncino Pentateuch, which has an English translation alongside the Hebrew text and an English summary of the classic Hebrew commentators. I brought him those books. Kashruth was another problem for him. I got him our kosher menu and talked to his dietician about extending to him every possible help. He moved around in a wheelchair in Housman 7 – Rehabilitation Unit, keeping his skullcap on.

I found out that he was a lonely man with no family to visit him. Good people from the Jewish community took an interest in him. And how surprised I was when I met a good-hearted religious lady in his room. She introduced herself as the person who had called me up a week before and asked for my help in having a crippled young man transferred from a city hospital to Mount Sinai for rehabilitation. I had instructed her how to proceed, and she thanked me for my guidance. The patient in the wheelchair was the patient I had helped come here! I was very glad to hear this.

English-Yiddish Index Cards

An elderly Romanian-Jewish immigrant could not relate to our staff because of a language barrier, and both his nurse and social worker asked for my help. At my suggestion, the nurse wrote all possible requests he might have on index cards, in English, and I added their Yiddish translation. This way, the patient, nurse, and social worker could use them as needed.

Inadequate Insurance Policy

A year and a half after I had been of some help to her in our psychiatry ward, she called for an appointment. The problem was her husband's inadequate medical insurance policy, issued to him by a yeshiva where he served in the Religious Department. It turned out that it covered only one month of psychiatric hospitalization while she had stayed two months. They were unable to pay some $10,000 – for the second month. The hospital had given the bill to a collection agency, as is common practice, and the agency was about to sue her. In despair, she and her husband came to solicit my help. I am very glad to state that after visiting a number of departments in our administration along with them, I was led to the office of the senior associate director, Social Work Services, who is resolving this case to the satisfaction of both the hospital and this couple.

Husband Does Not Want Her Back Home

A daughter of a patient asked for my intervention in not sending her ailing mother back to her second husband, who refused to take her in and might mistreat her. I brought this problem to the attention of a social worker, who subsequently met with the family and the husband, a Holocaust survivor and a difficult man to live with. The conclusion we reached was to find some accommodation for the patient outside her home, as her daughter had requested.

Seeking Proper Community

A physician completing his residency at our hospital approached me for guidance on how to find out if a community in which he would be interested to settle has the Jewish religious and cultural environment he needs and wants. I advised him to inquire from national rabbinic organizations the names of their members who serve such communities and then to contact those rabbis and visit them before he decides to settle there.

"I Have Been Readmitted. Please Come to See Me"

Former patients who return to our hospital for treatment or surgery call upon their readmission, asking that I see them again. During such visits, they usually relate their present medical problems as well as their fears. I offer them reassurance and the promise of frequent follow-up visits, especially after surgery. I sense this has a calming effect on them. They feel they are not alone. The rabbi whom they know from before will give them his special attention and care. Family members of former patients also call promptly, identifying themselves and asking for visits and extra attention. Patients certainly appreciate someone who cares.

"I Want to Live"

This middle-aged lady patient had undergone a mastectomy, following which the surgeon had informed her that he found no spreading of the disease in the vicinity of the operation. This gave her a measure of relief. Yet, deep inside her were fear and worry. She had singlehandedly raised two sons, one of whom was already a physician and the other in medical school, and she so much wanted to reap some happiness from her labors and struggles. "Why is this happening to me now?" she cried. "I want to live." She was so glad to have me visit with her, and we talked a long while about deposits of merits one makes in one's account in God's bank, drawings on those merits, making additional deposits, and trusting God. I left her calmed and relaxed, looking at life with greater hope and faith.

Being Old, Alone, and Helpless

When I introduced myself to her, she immediately responded that she was very distressed and wanted to talk to me. She had undergone a number of tests and two operations, felt weak and feared going home. She had been divorced, had no children, and lived alone. Given her age, status, and state of mind, being discharged from the hospital was a menace to her. I began by telling her that we do not just discharge patients. We feel it is our duty to determine if the patient is able to take care of herself at home. For that, our social service works out a regimen for the patient. In her case, it meant getting her a homemaker or a live-in companion. As she could not relate well to the social worker on her floor, I promised to get involved in her case till a satisfactory solution was reached. Of course, I first got in touch with her social worker, and a solution acceptable to the patient was worked out.

Another problem of hers involved a dispute with a private duty nurse on the number of hours the nurse had worked, and for which she wanted to get paid. To iron out this problem, I suggested that the nurse's report to the hospital be checked, as it is our practice to have such private nurses report to the hospital in written form.

Use of Authority to Benefit Patient

A young divorcee had a neurological problem, yet she insisted on discharging herself. She wanted to return to her two jobs in order to be close to and maintain the affection of her two children, who were temporarily being taken care of by their father. The physician and the private nurse voiced their opposition in my presence. I then firmly stated to her, "You are not leaving." I further explained to her the implications of her undoing whatever improvement was achieved. I also recommended that the children be brought to her once a week so as to diminish her fear of alienation. The patient consented and stayed another few weeks, during which time I checked on her medical progress and showed interest in her welfare. At the last meeting before her official medical discharge, she expressed her gratitude to me for my firmness with her and my personal interest in her well-being.

Troubled Patient

I found a troubled patient in an argument with his wife, who reprimanded him while their daughter stood nearby all forlorn. They advised me not to visit the patient because he was disturbed. But it was part of my job to visit "disturbed" patients. Sometimes a chaplain can empathize with a troubled man more quickly than a doctor. I told the family that, on the contrary, I wanted to speak to him. Fortunately, I managed to calm him down, answer his clamors for death, and make him regain his composure. A blood test was given to him in my presence and with his full cooperation. What happened was that his wife was too emotionally involved and exhausted to handle her sick husband successfully.

Hesitation Overcome

This patient told me that he was hesitant about undergoing surgery. Then he added that a son of his attended the Lubavitcher yeshiva. Whereupon I recommended that he consult the Lubavitcher Rebbe, one of the outstanding sages of our time. The patient felt relieved upon hearing this. He now had someone he knew and trusted to turn to for guidance.

"Rabbi, Do You Have a Minute?"

One of our nurses stopped me in the hall with the question, "Rabbi, do you have a minute?" She had a Hassidic patient on her maternity floor who, following a prolonged stay at our hospital with illness complicating her pregnancy, was ready to be discharged but needed someone reliable to guide her in her community and assist her in resolving upcoming problems. Our nurse suggested that I recommend an understanding lady from Bikur Cholim. Luckily, I knew such a person who also had a background in psychology. All elated, the nurse took the information which, she and staff felt, would extend a helping hand to this patient.

Comforting a Stroke Patient

Dear Director:

My husband was a stroke patient in the Rehabilitation Center for two months during the time of the Jewish holidays. I am writing to thank you for making available the services conducted by Rabbi Spirn which I attended with my husband and with other patients and their wives.

I'm also very grateful for Rabbi Spirn's visits to my husband throughout his stay at Mount Sinai. The few times I met Dr. Spirn, I was comforted by his compassion and intelligence. I know other wives of patients felt the same, so I want to say thank you for all of us.

Sincerely,

Is Minimum Improvement Sufficient for Discharge?

He was a Russian-Jewish immigrant who had undergone cardio-thoracic (open heart) and vascular surgery at our hospital. Just as he began walking, the physician discharged him. As he had no family and lived by himself, the social worker arranged for a visiting nurse and a home help aide to visit him a few times a week. However, he was frightened to go home when he could not walk well, and with tears in his eyes, he begged me to intervene. He wanted to stay a few more days.

I talked to his physician about holistic medicine, which is a religious concept as well: that while treating the illness, we also treat the patient, who is a suffering human being. In fact, newspapers recently reported from Boston that Harvard Medical School students have been directed to some courses in the humanities precisely for this purpose: to humanize their approach to the patient. Let us not rush a patient home when he had only a minimum of improvement.

I was about to have a few days of extension granted to this troubled patient when the physician visited him again and discovered a setback to this patient's recovery, a setback which later led to a third operation. The following words of the *Ethics of the Fathers* come to mind: "Wise men, be careful in your pronouncements." A little more humility is asked of all of us.

Letter from Patient's Husband

May 15, 1987

Dear Director:

My wife has recently completed a five-week stay at the Mount Sinai Hospital. I write to you to try to express to you in words our thanks and appreciation for your wonderful chaplain, Rabbi Charles Spirn.

I really wonder if Mt. Sinai realizes the great asset he represents to the patients. Watching him work day by day and Sabbath by Sabbath all these weeks, I really had to marvel how one man could accomplish so much. In any other hospital, you would need the services of at least three. Rarely have I ever seen such devotion and dedication on the part of an individual. I have to admire the way he personally identifies with the patients. He rejoices with them when they seem to be on the way to recovery and personally agonizes with them when they experience pain and discomfort. I have personally seen at services the faces of individuals etched with despair suddenly light up from the encouragement and prayers they received at the hands of Rabbi Spirn.

How fortunate we were to enjoy the services of such a remarkable person.

Gratefully yours,

9: SUPPORT AT POINT OF CRISIS

"Not Alone in Our Time of Need"

5 Sept. 1994

Dear Rabbi Spirn,

I just wanted to let you know how much your visits (and special prayers while I was in the surgical waiting room) meant to me during my daughter's stay in the hospital. Your thoughts were an inspiration to both of us during some dark and frightening hour. Thank God, my daughter had a good recovery and will soon go home. Thank you for being there and for reminding me that we are not alone in our time of need.

Wishing you a healthy and happy New Year from

Mother –

Enclosed: $100

Medical and Spiritual Healing Memorandum

To: Rabbi Dr. Charles A. Spirn, Head Chaplain
From: Dr. ---

Yesterday, I was one of the group of "congregant-patients" present at your enjoyable Sabbath services and sermon, and today I am at home ready to resume a normal mode of living once again. I send this note in appreciation of all the excellent care I received at the Mount Sinai Medical Center – and your moving "spiritual healing" completed the range of medical-nursing-food service: all of a caring and excellent quality.

Many thanks and appreciation to you.

Sincerely,
–, Ph.D.

Finding One's Roots

I had seen this patient in his room before surgery and later in the CCU.

I knew he was puzzled by his family name. How great was his surprise when I told him that his was the name of a great Talmudic scholar who had lived in Spain in the eleventh century and whose writings are studied regularly in any advanced yeshiva. At a later meeting I brought him two photocopied pages with biographical data about his ancestor, and he felt I had given him a most precious gift.

Religious Books at Morgue

When deceased persons are taken to the morgue, especially on Saturdays and Jewish holidays, family members wish to sit nearby and offer prayers till after sundown, when it is permissible to move the body to a funeral home. In order to accommodate such families, I have placed several items on the shelf of the morgue's waiting room: Hebrew-English books of Psalms, a book of Psalms in large-print Hebrew, a booklet entitled "Journey into the Night" and ten skullcaps. I also obtained permission from the Pathology Department, through the good offices of the morgue coordinator, to allow family members to stay in the morgue's waiting room throughout the day and night as well, thereby having the body watched continuously, and prayers offered continuously, in accordance with Jewish practice.

Jewish Divorce Problems

This year, in particular, both patients and staff turned to me with problems in Jewish divorce. The couples had already been granted the civil divorce but were unfamiliar with the proceedings for obtaining a Jewish divorce, a *get*. They were all given pertinent information and guidance in Jewish religious law on this subject and directed to a universally recognized rabbinic court called Beth Din. We thereby helped these people to close a painful chapter in their personal lives and directed them toward a better outlook for the future. The bride of a remarried man writes, "Thanks for all your help with our marriage plans."

Calling on Telephone on Purim?

From our optical dispensary came a surprising question: Can one call a religious person on the Purim festival? I responded that we are permitted to use electrical devices and even work on this festival because Purim is a semi-festival and is not one of the five major holidays which require abstaining from work. I nonetheless appreciated the caller's sensitivity and effort to make sure not to offend a religious person.

No Signature on Sabbath

A Jewish lady who was treated in our Emergency Room on Saturday had to be admitted to our hospital as an in-patient. For that, her signature was requested. She refused to comply due to religious constrictions on writing on the Sabbath. My intervention was requested. Since writing is prohibited on the Jewish Sabbath and holidays, I suggested that the patient declare that she is voluntarily checking herself into our hospital, with two staff members serving as witnesses. Then, on Saturday night or Sunday, she could sign the appropriate forms. The same principle is to be followed in our Psychiatry Department, when patients receive a pass to spend the day outdoors in the company of a relative. Similarly, thumb stamping (fingerprinting) is to be replaced by a declaration in front of two witnesses. The above procedure was accepted by our hospital. We are particularly grateful to the consultant in nursing, for her backing of this procedure, which avoids conflicts between religious Jewish patients and our administration.

Recites Psalm 130 in Tears

He was sitting in a chair, and, though the weather was relatively warm, he was wrapped in a blanket. He was an elderly man, visibly suffering. He asked me for a skullcap and then, with tears in his eyes, he recited Psalm 130 by heart in Hebrew: "Out of the depths have I cried unto Thee, O Lord. Hear my voice, O Lord, let Thine ears be attentive to the voice of my supplications..." I offered words of comfort to him, gave him recognition for his knowledge of Hebrew prayer and promised him an extra visit on the Sabbath. He wiped off the tears that were flowing on his cheeks and seemed to have regained his composure and a measure of peace of soul, if not peace of mind.

Repeating the Sermon Twice

She was a young married woman and attended our Sabbath services regularly, together with her mother who spent the day at her bedside. She was the daughter of a rabbi and found particular inspiration in our sermons. When, on one Saturday morning, she arrived late because of medical treatment, she asked me for a *dvar Torah*, a Torah message. I obliged and repeated the sermon I had given earlier. She was most appreciative.

"I Need a Volume of the Talmud"

This religious and learned patient wanted to borrow a specific tractate of the Talmud, and he contacted me for help. Fortunately, last year I had bought a twenty-volume set of the Talmud for our patient's library. Therefore, I referred the patient to that library, which lends out books. It was exactly what he needed, and he blessed me for providing books of serious study to educated patients.

Religion Can Help Prevent Suicide

In the psychiatry ward, an Orthodox young man attempted suicide. He was placed under twenty-four-hour watch. I befriended him and taught him what the Jewish religion says about suicide. Upon gaining his confidence, I made him take an oath that he would never try to shorten his own life. Our relationship was such that when he introduced me to a patient or to staff, he referred to me as "our rabbi."

"Please See Me Again"

I found her on a stretcher ready to go for surgery. I offered a prayer and said words of comfort. She was going to undergo a hysterectomy, she said, while her cancer in another part of her body was under control. She was visibly scared. "Everyone undergoing surgery is scared," I replied. "But with God's help, you will recover and return to your family. The rate of recovery here is very high. God, indeed, walks around in our hospital and heals our patients."

She answered with a request: "Please see me again."

"I will see you Friday morning at 9:00 A.M. Remember, we have a date Friday, and, with God's help, I expect you to show up. I am very strict about that." Her face lit up with a smile as she was wheeled into the elevator to the operating room.

Iranian Refugee Requests a Blessing

He was not a patient at our hospital and yet insisted on seeing me. I gave him an appointment. He was in good health but worried about his lack of success with people he met in New York. He craved understanding and friendship that would enable him to establish himself economically in this city. As a child, he recalled, Iranian rabbis would bless people, and subsequently, they did well in life. He wanted me to do the same for him. As we know, Hassidic rebbes (sages) are usually approached with such requests. Yet he insisted on my giving him my blessing, as another Iranian Jew had told him of a similar problem with which he had come to me, and he added that he felt my blessing brought him Divine help. I obliged then, gave him a blessing, promised to repeat the blessing for him at the Torah on the Sabbath and handed him a printed prayer text with the *Shema*. I advised him to recite that prayer every day. He left my office a contented man and asked permission to call me in the future.

Fond Remembrance of Hospital's Seder

Dear Rabbi Spirn,

Wishing you, your family and all the patients in the hospital a happy Passover. I'll never forget last Pesach when I was in the hospital and you conducted the Seder. It was the most wonderful thing for me to be able to attend it. Thank you for everything you have done and everything you are doing now.

I am enclosing a cassette of my film *I Miss the Sun* as a small token of appreciation for your kindness.

With warm regards,

Mother's Death?

She just could not witness her aged mother's suffering in the ICU. When she saw me making my visit to that unit, she promptly identified me and, in a tremulous voice, said to me, "Rabbi, I am a Jewish Orthodox person. I cannot take the terrible suffering of my mother any longer. Please give me permission to disconnect the life support equipment, so that she may die in peace. Her physician does not give her more than a few days of life anyway. I cannot take it any longer. Why make her suffer so much?"

I empathized with this lady's feelings and with her mother's pain. However, causing someone's death is a very serious matter, so I gave her two replies. First, I told her that our religion prohibits it, and since she is a religious person, she should abide by that. Moreover, I added a second reason, a psychological reason, for not disconnecting the life support. "Imagine that you do it, and your mother dies. In the beginning, you will feel that you did her a favor, you stopped her suffering. But a few months hence, the thought will come to you that your decision led to killing your mom and you may develop a feeling of guilt. Then you will tell yourself, 'Why did the chaplain not prevent me from doing that?' And, in your heart, you will also blame me. So, I want to protect you from future guilt and I tell you, 'No. Leave her life to God. Let Him decide. One day, you will be grateful to me for having advised you thus, and you will live with peace of mind.'"

The lady listened to me. Two days later, her mother died a natural death. And while mourning the passing of a dear mother, the devoted daughter could see that it was a decision from On High.

Saving a Life: "He Would Be Dead by Now, Had He Not Come Here"

He was a very seriously ill patient at another hospital. His family wanted him to be transferred to Mount Sinai to be under the care of a top specialist at our hospital. They contacted me and asked me to obtain the consent of our physician to accept him as his patient, which I succeeded in doing. Following the transfer, I visited that patient regularly. I was astonished two weeks later when the physician told me, "He would be dead by now, had he not come here." I surely felt gratified for having extended myself on behalf of that patient. And thank God for that good physician who was instrumental in saving a life.

"Do It for Me"

As I inquired about the well-being of this patient, the supervisor, who watched over her, told me that the patient had checked herself in only the day before and now wanted to check herself out. The physician treating her felt it was dangerous for her to check out, so the supervisor asked for my intervention. I soon discovered the nature of the illness (seizures) and the patient's plans to take a long trip overseas for professional reasons, while the physician was concerned about her ability even to walk out of the building. She was bright but headstrong and claimed she could always get medical and hospital attention overseas, too. Since no logical argument persuaded her, I asked her to do it for me, to stay because I advise it, and I promise to visit her daily to watch over her progress and to offer daily prayers for her recovery. To the surprise of the supervisor, the patient reacted positively to my request.

"This is a major breakthrough that you accomplished," the supervisor said, "and we are very grateful to you." In turn, I asked that whatever tests were to be given her be done without long delays, so as not to tax the patience of this patient.

I returned daily to see her. When she wavered at times on her commitment to stay, I advised the supervisor not to argue but just cut the patient's argument by stating, "You will have to discuss this with the rabbi." This approach worked. As I reminded her of her promise not to go home until the physician discharged her, she replied, "I give you my word." And let me add: She kept her word.

Helping Cardiac Patient and Staff

Following bypass heart surgery and a transfer to a regular room three days later, he could not breathe well because of water in a lung. The physicians recommended thoracentesis (aspiration of the fluid). Since he had to sign authorization for that procedure, he figured it was dangerous and declined it. When I visited him, he told me that he could not breathe for the second night, and therefore, he got out of bed and slept while sitting on a chair.

Upon inquiry, the staff told me that the fluid in the lining of one lung prevented the expansion of the lung, making it difficult for him to breathe. The Lasix pills seemed insufficient. Moreover, he ran the risk of developing an infection. Staff, including the surgery assistant, pleaded with me, asking me to win the patient's approval.

I decided to contact the patient's private physician, who had had him admitted to our hospital. As he too was urging the procedure be done, I asked him to make a telephone call to the patient, which he did immediately. Returning to the patient, I offered prayers for the success of the thoracentesis. The cardiac surgeon and his assistant then carried through the procedure successfully.

Caring for an Israeli Physician

Dear Director:

My husband (on sabbatical for one year from Israel) was operated on in your hospital on June 1. We would like to tell you that we were very much pleased by almost everything in the hospital, the doctors, nurses, the rest of the medical staff, but especially by the hospital's head chaplain, Rabbi Dr. Charles Spirn. He came to be with me while my husband was being operated on and gave me courage and fortitude. He came to see my husband every day, took care that he should get the kosher food he needed, and [attended to] his other religious needs. He gave us the feeling that we were not alone. There was someone who really cared for us.

Thank you,

"Why Couldn't My Doctor Talk Like You?"

She was very nervous; she was scheduled for open heart surgery in three days. I gave her reassurance. Moreover, I added, the rate of recovery in our cardiac unit was extremely high. "God must be walking around here and healing our patients," I said. I also told her where she would go after surgery and depicted all the steps till discharge, ten days after surgery. This calmed her greatly. In a more confident tone of voice, she then asked, "Why couldn't my doctor talk to me like you do?"

It was a good question. Why indeed? However, I gave this patient some excuses for why her doctor had not related better to her by giving her more time and offering more empathy and a ray of hope for recovery. Following surgery, I saw her twice in the Cardiac CU, and she was recuperating beautifully.

"I Am Glad You Are Here"

I had visited her mother when the daughter stopped me in the hall, saying that she had an important question for me. When I asked her what it was, she just replied, "I am glad you are here. Give me your card. I want to be able to call on you."

Twelve-Year-Old Thanks Rabbi

April 30, 1991

Dear Director:

I am a twelve-year-old girl whose mother has been at your hospital for almost three years now. At her side, mostly every day, was Rabbi Spirn...He was very supportive to my mother.... Rabbi Spirn helped my mother and my family through tough times. Just thought you should know Rabbi Spirn, head of the chaplains, is a very good rabbi and knows how to bring the best out of bad situations.

Thank you.
Sincerely,

Yiddish in English Alphabet for a Nurse

Seeing me on my rounds, this nurse asked me if I spoke Yiddish. She had an elderly Russian-Jewish patient who had undergone prostate surgery, and she could not communicate with him. I gladly served as the translator and then wrote two questions for the nurse to read in an English transliteration. The questions were: "Do you have pain?" "Where?" Our nurse pronounced the Yiddish very well.

"Helpful to Strangers in a Strange Town"

Chicago, Illinois
May 12, 1996

Dear Rabbi Spirn:

This letter is long overdue. I want to thank you on behalf of my husband and myself for the kindness and interest you showed us when my husband was a patient in our Cardiothoracic Surgical Intensive Care Unit in February after he was transferred to Mount Sinai from a Staten Island hospital. You were considerate and helpful when we were strangers in a strange town.

Thanks and best wishes.

Israeli Patient Follows Rabbi's Recommendation and Gets Well

After the family of an Israeli patient read my articles in an American-Jewish weekly newspaper, they contacted me for advice. The patient was suffering from ulcerated colitis. I recommended the chairman of our Gastrointestinal Department, since I know that he has regular contact with Israeli physicians and hospitals.

The patient came to us directly from the Hadassah Hospital in Jerusalem and received full medical attention and treatment. I also made arrangements for room and board for his young wife. I visited the patient regularly until he was discharged, luckily without needing surgery. The couple stayed on for ten days with another family and, after a final office visit and check-up with the physician, returned back home to Kiryat Arba for Passover. The complete family circle expressed gratitude for the personal attention I had given him in a beautiful letter to the editor printed in *The Jewish Press*.

A Difficult Patient?

One of our nurses called about a problem with a patient. He turned out to be a middle-aged Satmar Hassid, and our nursing staff were at their wit's end because he ignored their instructions as to walking and coughing, and he refused to be helped out of bed by female nurses. When I entered his room, I found him to be an intelligent man who was transacting business on a large scale with someone overseas via the telephone. When he stopped his lengthy long-distance call "because the rabbi of the hospital is in my room," we had a friendly conversation, after which I requested that he get out of bed and do some walking in the hall. He replied that he wanted to wait for the arrival of a male friend of his who would help him out of bed. Hearing this, I offered to give him a hand, which he hesitated to accept because of respect due to a rabbi. I quoted Talmudic law to him on this point and persuaded him to cooperate, which was a happy surprise to our nursing staff. In my presence, I had the nurse tell him what is required of him following his recent surgery in terms of walking, coughing, etc. I also asked that reasons be given to him for these requirements, such as the fear of his developing pneumonia if he does not do it. He accepted the explanation and, with the aid of two canes provided by the nurse, did his walking and promised to abide by medical advice.

The whole problem arose because he did not want female nurses to touch him. Yet he could have asked to be attended by a male nurse (male nurses are available at the hospital), but it did not occur to him to ask for one.

Assistance to Chaplains

Throughout the year, chaplains from many parts of the country continue to call or write for guidance in their work. I am glad to be able to provide information and counsel as well as share materials they can utilize in their work, such as copies of my annual report and samples of the programs of various functions that our chaplaincy organizes for our patients.

Israeli Guests on Friday Nights at Rabbi's Home

A man in his early thirties, veteran of the Yom Kippur War, was paralyzed from the chest down. He moved around in a wheelchair. His wife and brother-in-law accompanied him to America for treatment at our hospital. All three of them were my personal guests for the Sabbath meal on the few Friday nights that he got off. They were members of a nonreligious kibbutz in Israel. Before leaving this country, they requested a few of our booklets containing prayers such as *Kiddush* and Grace After Meals, as well as Sabbath songs which they enjoyed at my home. Our hospital did its very best for him.

Custodial Care or Rehabilitation? Rabbi's Suggestion is Followed

He was transferred to our psychiatric ward from another hospital, to which he had been taken after a suicide attempt: He had overdosed on pills. At that hospital, he had had cardiac arrest, which seemed to have affected the functioning of the brain through lack of oxygen. Our staff felt that the brain was organically damaged and, therefore, that the patient should be placed in a nursing facility. After half an hour's personal conversation, the patient opened up a bit and cried, and above all, talked and gave rational answers. It seemed to me that his family had a point when they hesitated to accept the suggestion that he be sent for custodial care in a nursing home for the rest of his life. I also felt an effort ought to be made to rehabilitate him.

At my suggestion, the family called another neurologist for consultation. Then, the Burke Institute screeners examined him, and felt their services would not be of help to him. So instead of rushing him to a nursing facility, he stayed on in our hospital and then, unexpectedly and slowly, he recuperated to the point where he was sufficiently well-functioning to be discharged and continue as an outpatient in a hospital near his home. Throughout his stay, I was in touch with him and his family and brought relief to them all, but particularly to him, because his confidence in me led us to discuss the problem which led him to suicide in the first place.

Only Two Visitors at a Time

The nursing station of AICU called to ask for my intervention with a Hassidic patient in their unit whose little room was filled with visitors. They requested that I persuade the family to have only two visitors at a time. I obliged, and the problem was soon resolved in a friendly way. I explained to the family that having a crowd in a small room puts a strain on the patient and on other patients. In fact, most of the time, there is no need for radical measures to enforce patients' observance of hospital regulations. I appreciate having been called first. I usually resolve such problems in a peaceful way.

Uproar in Emergency Unit

A nurse from the emergency unit's surgical department called urgently: A Jewish lady had requested the rabbi. It turned out that the lady was in pain, caused by the accidental laceration of her leg. While a bag of ice was applied to her wound, she insisted on being treated without delay and voiced her woes in a loud voice. There was no way to calm her down, as she imagined her condition to be very grave. Realizing that, I approached a surgeon and asked him to please handle this case first. The surgeon cleaned the wound, gave her a local anesthesia to numb the area of the cut, and stitched the skin. All the while, the patient, nervous and uncontrollable, held my hand for emotional support. She was a widow living by herself and had neither family nor close friends. She poured out to us the bitterness of her situation. With the leg finally bandaged she was able to walk and took a taxi to her home. I had spent an hour and a half on this case. I do realize that without my intervention, this problem, compounded by uncontrolled emotional outbursts, could not have been handled constructively.

On Verge of Discharging Herself

She was an elderly lady with a physical illness, inconsolable about the passing of her husband, which led her to a depression. When I entered her room, she was getting ready to leave after a stay of two weeks. The nurse who assisted her kept on telling her that she should not discharge herself, but she would not listen. She had no children, lived by herself, and felt that she would manage at home by getting a helper. I called her attention to the present need for medical attention, something she would not get at home, and urged her to stay a few more days as her physician suggested. It took me some time to persuade her to stay, but she finally consented. In reaction to her complaint about spending all her time in bed or on a chair next to it, I recommended that she be brought to our Saturday morning services in a wheelchair and have a change of scenery and atmosphere. The staff and I were pleased by her change of heart.

Physician as a Son

As I entered my office in the morning, the telephone rang. A physician called, urging me to please see his mother, a patient at our hospital, forthwith as she was scheduled to go for surgery in five minutes. I did manage to see his mother and offered a prayer on her behalf and gave comfort to her. She had eye surgery, and I saw her again after the operation. Her son was in constant touch with her by phone. His devotion to her, she told me, was beyond description.

Responding to Israeli Family

Weeks before their arrival from Israel, I was briefed that these parents would bring their teenage child for brain surgery at our hospital. We managed to find sleeping quarters for the couple. I am also particularly grateful to the administrator of Support Services for responding to my request and ordering free daily breakfasts and lunches, while the Satmar Women's Bikur Cholim brought daily dinners. We also provided the family with other equipment to make their stay as pleasant as possible. I am very glad to say that surgery was successful and that the family left our hospital with the feeling that we all did them much good.

Prompt Communication and Translation

Since this Jewish psychiatric patient spoke little English, the supervisory nurse did not understand what she was complaining about and called me up to serve as the translator. I recommended that the nurse give the patient the phone so that I could talk with her in Yiddish, and then take the receiver herself to get my translation. The three-way conversation worked out well and, within minutes, the supervisor knew what irked the patient. The problem – nausea – was related to the patient's treatment, and the nurse knew what could make her feel better.

Tolerance of Pain

This patient moaned and groaned aloud, saying that his pain was unbearable. His roommates, however, felt that he was exaggerating, and therefore they deprecated him. My reaction was to call in his nurse and ask for her help. At the same time, I offered him comfort. Then I explained to his roommates that the level of tolerance of pain varies between people and that we must have sympathy and give relief to people in pain, even if it is subjective.

"You Are a Godsend to Us"

The patient was in surgery for cancer, and his large family was waiting in his room. They were out-of-town Sabbath-observing people, and it was the Friday before the Sabbath of Repentance and four days before Yom Kippur. I helped take care of the family's needs.

First, they needed a few rooms near the hospital to sleep over Friday night and the eve of Yom Kippur. This was resolved by having the family rent rooms in our new Jane B. Aron Residence Hall. The next problem was candelabra with eight branches (lights) for use by four women. A Hanukkah menorah took care of that. The third problem was food. I got them some, especially for immediate use and for the Sabbath, from our kitchen, and then connected them with the dietician of their floor, from whom visitors may order kosher meals.

Finally, the surgeon stepped in and reported on the operation, which was successful as far as he could determine. However, possible chemotherapy and life expectancy remained to be seen. For the near future, though, there seemed to be no danger. A united and grateful family then expressed heartfelt thanks for my words of comfort and added, "You are a Godsend to us."

Talking Out His Options Helps Him Make a Decision

A lonely patient, a librarian in one of our metropolitan colleges, underwent heart bypass surgery. Now he was uncertain whether to return to his position or to go to his sister in Florida. He was happy, indeed, to have me listen to him as he talked out the pros and cons of each possibility, and we arrived at what we considered the best decision in this case.

Revenge?

In our ACCU, I found a cardiac patient who took ill after aggravation with a person he had taken into his business. She had somehow mishandled his finances. However, he had no legal proof that she did. He asked me if he should avenge himself since he had a way of doing her harm. My advice: not to do it. If he cannot take her to a civil court, the case will go to the Court on High. Leave the matter to Heaven. She may still regret her act and at least ask forgiveness. The patient cheered up, accepted my advice, and relaxed, his anger largely dissipated.

Calling Personal Rabbis of Patients

A depressed lady spoke fondly of her rabbi, whom she had known for a few decades. I contacted him, and he had a telephone conversation with her. Another patient, who had been in a wartime concentration camp, expressed his strong desire to see again the Jewish chaplain who helped in his liberation. Here too I contacted the rabbi who paid a visit to our patient and cheered him up.

Death Wish Overcome

A nurse had me paged to handle the case of a depressed lady who wanted to die. She had lost her husband and a daughter within a short span of time and talked of joining them.

Following my introduction, the patient received me cheerfully and with a big smile. I congratulated her on her cheerfulness. After an exchange of niceties, I successfully had her sip milk and soda to prevent dehydration, which was also a major problem for her. At the end of my visit, which I promised to repeat on the following days and did, her surviving daughter, a psychotherapist, remarked, "You have done very well, Rabbi. Thank you."

10: IN THE VALLEY OF THE SHADOW

Unburdens Before Chaplain

She was a married woman in her early thirties. Two members of her family held her, one under each arm, while she kept crying bitterly in one of the halls of our hospital. As I passed that hall, I walked in the direction of the crying and was immediately briefed: Her husband had had surgery, and the physician had just told her that the cancer was widespread in his abdomen. I had seen the woman at her husband's bedside in the dialysis section, and the next day I paid them a visit. Both were glad to see me.

I invited the lady into the hall so we could talk openly without disturbing her sick husband. We sat side by side on a bench, and I encouraged her to verbalize her feelings of distress. This couple had been dealing with illness for a year. They had gone to Pittsburgh for a liver transplant, which was extremely expensive, and were collecting money from insurance and private donations to cover it. They thought that they had overcome the illness, when he suddenly got sick again. On the operating table, the surgeon discovered that the cancer had spread and would require chemotherapy.

I tried to offer some comfort to this heartbroken wife and mother of two. Slowly, the woman regained her composure and returned to her husband's room with some ray of hope and the will to do everything necessary to save his life. However, before chemotherapy could begin, he took a turn for the worse and returned his soul to its Divine Maker.

Alone and Fearful

She was very glad to see me when I introduced myself for the first time. Soon, however, she burst out crying. The reason: She was afraid she had cancer of the liver, although she had no basis for that fear. The physician had only begun his search for diagnosis. I remained with her for a long while, and we chatted. She was the alarmist type, going to extremes and imagining the worst. I succeeded in calming her fears and visited her frequently. Finally, her diagnosis was established. It was not at all life threatening, as she had feared, and she was going to be discharged. She became tearful again during my last visit – this time, she said, in recollection of our previous encounters. In bidding her good-bye, I said, "May God keep you well and also teach you how to smile." I think I saw the beginning of a smile.

11:00 P.M. Confession

An emergency call at 11:00 P.M. by the assistant director brought me to the bedside of a middle-aged patient who was considered terminal. I had befriended him during his long stays at our hospital, and he always cheered up in my presence. This time, however, he was asleep, and his sister and niece were with him. They had insisted on my being contacted, and I am glad that the assistant director obliged. I recited the last Confession (*Viduy*) for him and continued with the prayer for the dying. In the quiet of the night at the hospital, I softly recited the words of prayer, "May it be Your will to send perfect healing to him. Yet, if You have decreed that he be taken by death, let it be in love. May his death atone for the shortcomings committed before You. Grant him shelter in the shadow of Your Presence and let him merit resurrection.... Hear, O Israel, the Lord is our God, the Lord is one...." He remained alive for some additional two weeks, during which I visited him often and spoke to his devoted family. Then, he succumbed to the slumber, the awakening from which is in the Hands of God alone.

Crisis: Stays Day and Night at His Brother's ICU

This rabbinic patient underwent heart bypass surgery, and suddenly his condition became aggravated. His wife and his children came over, and his brother flew in from out of town with his family. They had all spent the night in the waiting room and hall of Annenberg 8, near the CCU. As the family insisted on remaining close to the patient, I obtained kosher milk, cereal, grape juice, and bananas from our kosher kitchen for that family circle in need. The next day, Friday, was Martin Luther King's birthday. Since they insisted on spending that Friday night (the Jewish Sabbath) in the hall, I obtained permission from the administrator and from our Security Department for the family to use the Exercise Room near the CCU on that legal holiday. Three cots were placed therein for rest. Two family members from out-of-town were guests at my home for the Sabbath eve meal and sleeping accommodations. I visited the patient very frequently. Unfortunately, the patient did not make it.

The patient's brother, a noted rabbinic and academic personality, wrote: "I know what our sages have taught, that rewards for good deeds are not often given in this world, but an expression of thanks for your genuine kindness, hospitality, and assistance is certainly in order. Your benevolence transcends the requirements of your position. We shall always remember your help at an extremely difficult time."

"Say *Shema* with Me"

He stood near his bed when I came over and introduced myself. When he heard that I was a rabbi, his very first words to me were, "Say *Shema* with me." I handed him the text of the *Shema* from one of our prayer cards and gave him a skullcap to cover his head. And so, standing side by side with him, I was witness to his praying the most important prayer in the Jewish religion in Hebrew, proclaiming the unity of God and our duty to love Him with all our heart, with all our soul, and with all our might. Tears kept running down his face as, in fairly fluent Hebrew, he recited the *Shema* and the following prayers printed on that card. I admired the depth of his religious feelings and the comfort prayer brought to him.

A Death on Yom Kippur

A staff member of the hospital's Security Department knocked at my door in the middle of the night. A Jewish patient had died and I was needed. It turned out that a daughter of the deceased was frail, frightened, and alone and was at a loss on what to do. Ideally, since the deceased occupied a private room, she could remain there. However, the supervisor and the night administrator felt that it was a long stretch of some twenty hours till the High Holy Day was over and the body could be removed. Moreover, it might start decomposing and, in addition, the bed might be needed for another patient. So the morgue became the solution.

In this sad situation, a helpful staff member knocked and slipped a note under the door of the Bikur Cholim apartment, explaining that the dead man's daughter-in-law who slept there should come urgently to the hospital. Mercifully, another couple who slept there accompanied her to the hospital floor so the two women could be together and give comfort to each other.

When the body was finally removed to the morgue, we all accompanied it, and then the two mourners were kept company by the kind couple who had been in the Bikur Cholim apartment. Only two hours later I returned home. In the early morning, at the neighborhood synagogue, I spoke to the Congregation Orach Chaim on Lexington Avenue, and they kindly arranged a team of ten volunteers to watch over the deceased at the morgue, one hour each. This proved to be a tremendous relief to the mourners, who participated in our chapel's services and then followed my advice to take some rest in the Bikur Cholim unit while volunteers from the congregation took turns at the morgue.

Of special help during these proceedings was our Security Department, which handled the numerous telephone calls needed to treat the deceased respectfully and bring some relief to the two bereaved women on this holiest night and day in the Jewish calendar. At the conclusion of Yom Kippur, I further helped the family contact a funeral director and have him remove the body from the hospital morgue.

Three Months to Live?

Her physician had told her that very morning that there was nothing more that he could do for her. She had ovarian cancer and had three months to live. As she talked, tears welled in her eyes. I was surprised that the doctor had revealed the sad news to her. She asked me how to cope with such a verdict. I let her talk about her marriage, which was a very happy one, about her two children, who were grown up and happily married, and about her aged mother, who lived in her vicinity. She particularly wanted to see a child from her daughter, who had had a miscarriage. I told her that the physician could only make an educated guess, for life is in the Hands of God alone, and He had been good to her. I brought her an example of a recent case I had, when the patient lived seventeen months and had gone back to work, though his doctor had given him only three months to live. And so, I encouraged her to pray to God to extend her life so she could see the birth of a grandchild. At the end of the visits, she said, "Thank you for having come at the right time."

Dealing with the Medical Examiner on Autopsy

She was seventy-six years old and underwent a right-above-knee amputation. She had a history of cardiac problems and was unstable throughout the procedure. Then, in the recovery room, she expired. I was immediately paged. Upon arrival, I was informed that the Medical Examiner's Office had been contacted, as protocol requires notifying them of the death of any patient during the first twenty-four hours post surgery. The patient had left a signed statement that her amputated leg be returned for burial as required by Jewish law. Her only relative, a niece, had also asked that the body be returned for prompt burial. The hospital, however, had to wait for a return call from the medical examiner, who, after a delay of a few hours, decided to have the body moved to his quarters.

Sadly, the deceased had left no family except the niece, whom I could not reach. That fact made my intervention more urgent. (It brought to mind the case of the ancient Jewish High Priest who purified himself in order to perform the Yom Kippur atonement service in the Temple. Yet Jewish law stipulates that if he finds a corpse in the field and there is no one else to take care of it, he must handle it, even though in the process he becomes impure and disqualified for the Temple service on the holiest of days. This Jewish law alerts us in no uncertain terms as to the prime value Judaism attaches to human dignity, as typified even by an unknown corpse on the road.)

Therefore, following consultation with COLPA, the legal branch of the Orthodox Union, I decided to contact the Medical Examiner's Office, where the deceased had already become a case number. I asked that, as head chaplain of our hospital, I be listed as voicing a religious objection to the autopsy of this patient. Upon talking further with their medical staff, I got them to drop the autopsy. The niece could come and identify her aunt and receive the proper papers authorizing removal of the body for religious burial. May the poor lonely lady rest in peace.

Battered Wife

We thought that this type of problem does not exist in Jewish life, yet it comes up from time to time. I knocked on this patient's door even though the sign said, "No visitors allowed." As it turned out, I was heartily welcomed: The patient felt she could best discuss what was on her mind with a rabbi. Her husband had thrown her against a chair, causing dizziness and bruises in her head. There was bone damage and bleeding. The cuts needed sutures, and she had to be hospitalized. Because of her husband's violence, she was now considering divorce. There seemed to be no chance of reconciling this couple. I then helped to raise her spirits and recommend she postpone a final decision till after her recuperation. In the meantime, she should continue her treatment in the hospital and contact family and friends to find a place where she could stay after her release, and there make a decision that is best for her.

Breathing Naturally or Only Through Respirator?

An emergency call from a nurse requested that I come immediately to be with the family of a dying patient. The family was very religious and hesitated to accept the patient's demise, as it looked like she was still breathing. Therefore, I asked the physician to examine the patient again and to tell us whether the patient had really expired and the breathing was due only to the respiratory machine. I asked whether he was 100 percent sure that death had occurred, or only 99 percent. In response, he suggested that we give the patient more time before reaching a conclusion.

In such a case, I guided the husband who had asked me whether he is permitted to don his prayer shawl (tallith) and phylacteries and pray the morning services. Since it was not certain that death had occurred at that point, formal prayer was still permissible. A nurse who had stepped in also concluded that the heart beat no longer, and it was the respirator alone that was giving the impression of the patient breathing. However, we waited for the physician's pronouncement. When he came in again, he clearly pronounced the patient dead, this time being completely sure. I then instructed the husband that religious law exempts him from completing the full morning prayers in order to take care of preparation for burial of his wife. He became an *onan*, I informed him, the status of family members from the time death is pronounced till after the interment, when one becomes an *ovayl*, a mourner. I then directed the family to call the funeral director of their choice and gather the belongings of the patient and her husband, who had spent this Passover weekend with his wife and had conducted the Seder in her room.

While the menfolk of the family were occupied with the preparation of the funeral, which they scheduled for that very afternoon, two daughters of the deceased broke out in terrible grief at the loss of their middle-aged mother. We took them into the floor's TV room, where they could express their pain and grief without upsetting the other patients on the floor. And there, I admired the brilliant cancer specialist who had treated the patient and now answered some of the daughters' questions. He stood and listened attentively and sympathetically to their expressions of admiration and love for their mother. While time is at a premium for this physician, he gave of it generously in order to achieve some release of this family's grief. I then encouraged the daughters to return home and prepare for the funeral. Their father expressed profuse thanks to me for my personal and religious ministrations to him and his family.

Twice in One Night at the Hospital

This happened on the Jewish Sabbath, Friday night, September 21, two days before Yom Kippur. At 2:00 A.M., a security guard knocked at my door and told me I was urgently needed in the hospital as a patient had died, and the family requested that I come. I hastened to reach the bereaved, prayed a Psalm at the bedside of the deceased, answered the family's questions, offered sympathy, and guided the religious mourners on how to proceed during the Sabbath. I then walked home.

Surprisingly, at 5:00 A.M., the same security guard knocked at my door again: Another Jewish patient had died in the CCU, and this family also requested I come. It was a family of Russian immigrants who were in shock at the passing of a middle-aged sister. I again offered a prayer in Hebrew and English and spent time bringing a measure of solace to this distraught family circle. As I left the hospital in the early hours of the morning, I prayed for Divine mercy for all the sick.

Finding Record of Time of Death

His childless aunt died at our hospital some eight months ago toward the evening. However, he was not sure if she died before or after sunset, which would affect the Hebrew date of her yahrzeit, the anniversary of her death, on which date special prayers, including kaddish, are to be recited for her. He had misplaced the death certificate and somehow could not reach the funeral director. Therefore, he turned to our hospital, which referred him to me. I am glad to state that I contacted our Medical Records Department and, to my pleasant surprise, received an answer promptly. The nephew felt a great sense of relief. Since death had occurred some forty-five minutes after sunset, the Hebrew date would then be the next day. It happened to be the first of Adar. As the present Hebrew year, 5746, was a leap year with Adar I and Adar II, I told the nephew to observe the yahrzeit twice in leap years, which occur seven times in nineteen years to reconcile the Jewish lunar calendar with the solar calendar.

"You Were Right There When We Needed You"

November 21, 1994

Dear Rabbi Spirn:

I have enclosed a donation to be used for furthering Jewish awareness at Mount Sinai, in honor of my dear wife.

The entire family wishes to express its gratitude to you for the efforts you made during her illness, which lasted approximately fifteen months. She appreciated and felt comforted by your visits to her room while she was in the hospital; especially when you would bring her the Shabbos candelabra on Friday. On Sukkoth, we enjoyed the mitzvoth of lulav and ethrog when you brought them to us for the proper prayers; of course, eating in the lovely sukkah at the hospital made it comfortable for me and my daughter.

You helped me very much by "showing me the ropes," i.e., telling me about the Orach Chaim synagogue nearby and showing me the beautiful chapel in the Guggenheim building. These sanctuaries helped us greatly in our hour of need. We had a place to pray in peace and quiet. Of course, introducing us to the Bikur Cholim apartment was of utmost importance.

At the end, you were right there when we needed you. My dear wife passed away on Shabbat, October 29, 1994. Your being there was a great comfort in that we knew we were doing everything correctly and according to Halakhah, in the utmost respect to our departed loved one.

May God give you strength to keep up the good work you are doing in keeping yiddishkeit strong.

Sincerely,

Enclosed: $100

A Frightened Patient

He had never been hospitalized before. In the hospital now at an advanced age, he insisted that his wife stay at his side constantly, fearing even to go for tests without her. Almost like a child, he was also adamant about "going home." His wife was at her wits' end in handling him when I came in for a visit.

We spent considerable time together chatting in Yiddish, in which he was more fluent than in English, though he had come to this country before the Second World War. He had some Jewish background while his wife had very little of it, except the language – Yiddish. He enjoyed my company and felt at ease with me. He also asked questions about Divinity and the Holocaust, in which his parents were killed. When we came to his resolve to check himself out, he listened attentively to my description of his prospective condition at home, where he would have neither a physician to see him daily nor the instruments for tests and medication. I advised him to be patient and promised additional visits. Though not formally religious, he acquiesced to my praying for him and gave me his and his mother's Hebrew names for use in prayers for recovery. On return visits, I found he had followed my advice to remain in the hospital and was progressing on his way to a cure.

Domestic Trouble

When I first visited this patient, he was in the middle of a telephone conversation and requested that I please come back the next day, as he had a serious problem to discuss. The problem turned out to be a domestic one, a long-lasting conflict and incompatibility with his wife, who had been suffering from a psychological illness and had received treatment for it. They also occupied separate sleeping rooms, and she locked hers at night. Their adult children were caught up in a quandary and tried hard to be of service to both parents. As he related incident after incident about his troubled life, he dozed off out of tiredness. Therefore, I promised to return to him the next day.

This time, he was alert and listened carefully to my advice. I gave him a two-point program. One was to have his local rabbi attend a meeting with the full family present and work out a plan that would be binding on all.

And secondly, he, our patient, should himself make an appointment with the Jewish Family Service and then request that he be given weekly or biweekly sessions with a social worker. I explained to him that such sessions would bring him relief, as they would provide him with a verbal and emotional catharsis instead of letting grievances accumulate inside him and undermine his fragile health. I must say that my advice pleased him enormously and raised his hope for long-needed relief.

Sudden Widowhood

On a Saturday morning, as I arrived to lead services, a nurse brought me a lady in tears. Her husband had undergone minor surgery and was recuperating at our Falk ICU when suddenly, at dawn, his heart gave way. He did have a long-standing heart condition, but his wife felt totally shocked and helpless. I directed her to our nearest congregation, Orach Chaim, on Lexington Avenue, where she found volunteers to take turns reciting Psalms at the door of the morgue. I also promised to come for her at lunchtime. I found her again tearful and disconsolate and invited her to my home to have the Sabbath meal with us, following which I insisted on her getting some sleep. In the evening, at the conclusion of the Sabbath, I made calls for her to her immediate family, including a daughter in the Catskills, as well as to the Jewish Sacred Society, which had to remove the body. Her friends and family members gathered in my home and managed to arrange transportation by 11:30 P.M.

Dying of Hunger?

Following our Sabbath morning services, I usually make some extra visits with some KCC patients. Suddenly, a private nurse who recognized me asked me to please see her patient immediately, as there was an urgent and most serious problem with him. When I entered the room, the patient's wife lamented over the fact that her ninety-two-year-old husband had not eaten and also had not been given intravenous feeding and was, therefore, dying of hunger and dehydration, and not out of illness as the physicians had told her. Upon inquiry, I learned that, indeed, the patient was considered terminal and staff relied on a resident's visit that morning. I requested to see the supervisor, but she was not on the floor. In the meantime, the patient's wife became hysterical, claiming again that we were letting her husband die of starvation and demanding that we get help fast. Continuing the search for the supervisor, one nurse somehow managed to find her. I then explained to her the urgency of the case and the possible immediate danger to his life. Her response was that this required the presentation of the case to the patient's physician. Luckily, as if by telepathy, the physician appeared. He examined the patient and found that he still had lots of fluid in his system, yet he reinstated him on IV, to the wife's satisfaction. Result: I followed up the case, and the patient was kept alive for a month.

Fear and Worry Changed into Hope and Confidence

Her nurse called me up, asking for a visit as the patient was very depressed, and her condition was regarded as serious. She had also remembered me from a previous stay at our hospital. She was a woman of great courage, but her illness had worn her down. "I cannot come to terms with death," she said. She was particularly worried about her two daughters, both collegians. As she talked about them, tears came to her eyes, and her lower lip trembled. I let her talk for a long while, giving her an opportunity to unburden herself. The thought that she might die soon and that her daughters would remain helpless troubled her enormously. Her husband, who sat at her bedside, added that there was a close, warm relationship between mother and children, and that she always resolved her children's problems and was a source of strength to them.

Following a long period of listening, I began by encouraging her to do everything possible to prolong her life. Fighting illness and struggling to overcome it is a Jewish religious command, I told her. While she does that with the help of her physician, all of us, referring to her, her husband, her children, and I, will pray for extension of life. Now, concerning her children, I pointed out that, due to her success as a mother, the daughters have internalized her strength, courage, and way of solving problems, so that she will always be present in their inner selves and continue to offer guidance to them. Then, their father is here to offer help and support, and the children themselves are growing into adulthood, independence, and professions. All that points to the ability to face life and not to fall. When a daughter called from school in my presence, I asked for the receiver. In her parents' hearing, I praised the daughter for her love and devotion, encouraged her to pray for her mother, congratulated her for doing well in her studies and for preparing well for a profession. I expressed my deep confidence in her ability to face life, as she was the daughter of a very capable and courageous mother whom she had seen in action. The talk to the patient and her daughter produced a more relaxed atmosphere with rays of hope and confidence in the future.

"I Must Talk to a Rabbi"

It was a Sunday morning when the nursing coordinator called me at home and asked me what to do about an outsider who telephoned our hospital and expressed her urgent need to talk to a rabbi. I decided to take the caller's phone number and return the call myself.

It turned out to be a lonely Jewish adult who tearfully poured out the bitterness of her heart to me. She had given up her apartment and moved in with her mother, in order to be near her during the terminal stage of her mother's illness, but her mother asked her to leave. A married sister of hers was handling the mother, together with a physician and a social worker, but wanted her neither to call nor to come over. In addition, according to my interlocutor, the married sister had the mother give over all her assets to her, the married sister.

During more than an hour's conversation, I succeeded in dispelling her guilt about not being able to see her mother in the last phase of her mother's life. She had a lifetime of honor and devotion to her mother on her record, and that is what counts. Moreover, her sister should be given the benefit of the doubt for keeping her away since she was a very emotional person, and it was hard enough for the sister and her husband to care for a terminal patient. I encouraged her to find herself a decent apartment. As she had no savings, I gave her the names of two charitable ladies of Bikur Cholim, who might lend her money for one month's rent and a month's security. Concerning the fear of being deprived of her share in her mother's inheritance by her sister, I gave her some relevant advice in case of need. "You did a lot for me," she concluded. "I needed a rabbi to help me survive this day."

Recommendation for Disability Coverage

This Iranian-Jewish young man had been a frequent outpatient in our Neurology Department following brain surgery performed on him in Iran. He was poor, without parents here, and unable to handle a job. His social worker applied for disability for him; however, to back up the application, a letter from our Neurology Department was needed. Since the physician who had treated him was no longer in charge, our refugee had a very hard time obtaining such a letter. Upset and in despair, for the nth time, he called on me for help. I did manage to put today's physician in touch with the physician who had treated this patient before for an extended period of time. The supervisor, whom I had interested in this case, later showed me the text of the official letter written by the new physician on the basis of the patient's chart and the conversation with the previous physician. I found it incomplete as it omitted the main point, the recommendation to grant him disability insurance. Wishing to protect the physician and yet help the patient, I had the physician add a sentence stating that *in his estimation*, the patient should be accepted for disability payments. This finally resolved the problem to everyone's satisfaction.

11: GRIEF

Help and Guidance at Time of Deep Grief

"Your support is urgently needed," was the message on my voice mail when I arrived at my office in the morning. Though it was the day before Yom Kippur, I changed my plans and rushed to the floor where the problem existed. The patient had died, and her husband was in shock. He was lying on a makeshift bed in the waiting room. This was an elderly childless couple, very attached to each other. He was a scholar and a teacher in a seminary. I let him express his deep grief at his loss. He knew me from this couple's previous stays at our hospital. He was so overwhelmed by what happened that he kept repeating that he wished himself dead. I turned the conversation to the question of what his wife would have told him at this time if she were in a position to speak. He agreed with me that she would have urged him to take good care of himself and continue his scholarship. In spite of his refusal to eat, I ordered a kosher breakfast for him. Then I outlined the steps to be taken, as his wife had wanted to be buried in Jerusalem. It so happened that I gained much information on this topic just a few months before, when I had taken a deceased member of our own family to Israel for burial.

I advised him to have the body removed to a funeral parlor that specializes in this type of service and schedule the funeral on the day following Yom Kippur at the New York chapel rather than have the main service in Israel. This would enable colleagues, friends, and students to attend and pay their last respects to his wife, instead of traveling to a new country where they had few acquaintances. Also, there would be little time on arrival on an early Friday afternoon to do anything more than a rather hurried burial service at the cemetery. Of course, travel arrangements also had to be made for the husband and a sister-in-law. I repeated this outline and left only after a friend of his arrived. I later checked again and found that my outline had proved helpful and was followed. At the husband's request, I contacted his seminary.

Later, an official representative of the school called me to express the faculty's deep gratitude for the help and guidance given to one of its scholars at a delicate and painful time.

Hassidim Also Need Chaplain's Guidance

An emergency call on my beeper brought me to our RCCU. Two Hassidic adult brothers, whose father's condition was considered critical, had called. They wanted to know the religious ruling about what to do right now, and what to do at the time of death and afterward.

I told them I was an Orthodox Rabbi, which put them at ease. I then gave the required information and instructions, including prayer texts to be recited at the time of death. While knowledgeable in Jewish learning, they had less familiarity with the practical Halakhah, the applicable law. I then offered Psalm 130 at the bedside of their aged, rabbinic father, who seemed to be asleep or in a coma. Yet he suddenly opened his eyes and his look, so full of wisdom, indicated he was aware of my prayer for God's compassion to him.

The rabbinic patient rallied eventually, and, following a few weeks of treatment during which he and his wife welcomed my regular visits, he was discharged. Indeed, a typical example of the Talmudic adage that even in the most stressful situations, while there still is a glimmer of hope, one should not despair of Divine mercy.

Yes Wig, No Wig

The husband of a psychiatric patient made a special request that I visit her. The psychiatrist, he told me, tried to reconcile them and prevent a divorce, but he felt his wife to be insufficiently religious because of her reluctance to wear a wig at all times. I saw the patient, a young woman, mother of two infants, who had tried suicide unsuccessfully. I worked out an agreement between the couple as to the occasions when the wig would be worn, and when a hat or other head covering would do.

He also complained that she had told him that she did not believe in God, and, therefore, he went back to the idea of divorce. I then made it clear to him that, in my observation, she was a completely religious person but her statement to him was just like throwing a book at him, to shock him and get even for what she felt was his mistreatment of her.

She strongly asserted her independence. She had been married at nineteen and had now matured; she wanted to lead her own style of life with no wig, freedom to wear pants when she wanted to, and general freedom to "do her own thing" within the framework of religion. She had also made peace with the fact that her husband would get their two children. Her physician felt that she was manic-depressive.

This case became complicated when she returned the marriage ring to her husband, insisting on a divorce and making plans to return to a relative's house and seek employment. All we could do was tell her that since divorce court proceedings take at least a year, she would be able to reevaluate her decision during that time and possibly reconsider. She attended our services and, upon discharge, thanked me profusely for helping in her recovery. I gave her my card for mail or phone communication.

Finds Repentance Impossible

This man, who had received a full Jewish education in his youth, now tortured himself for having abandoned God, he said, and having set a bad example for his son, an only child, whom he had raised alone after the early death of his wife. He had sent his son to a top Jewish Day School but that religious education proved to be of no avail, the father said, because he himself had not lived as a "practicing Jew." During his stay in our psychiatric ward, he would insist on his guilt, decline to return to religion as too late for him, and moan about the imminence of his death. I learned from his nurse that he also suffered from leukemia. I spoke to him of Divine forgiveness and did my best to bring some measure of comfort and friendship to his tortured soul till his discharge from our hospital.

Finding Hebrew Dates of Yahrzeit

Both patients and staff often ask me to find the Hebrew date corresponding to the English date of the passing of a close relative so that they may observe the anniversary (yahrzeit) at the right time. I find it for them in special multi-calendars. This puts their minds at ease, as it gives them the feeling that they are honoring the memory of their beloved properly by observing the yahrzeit through reciting kaddish, lighting a memorial lamp, and having the memorial prayer said at the Torah on the correct Hebrew date.

Teaches Inspirational Verses to Roommates

A patient who attended our Saturday services felt especially uplifted by the concluding hymn of the service, "*Adon Olam.*" She memorized the last lines, and the next time I visited her, she and her roommates recited those verses in unison. She had taught it to them, and they all gained strength and solace from those verses. The hymn describes God as Omnipotent Creator and loving Providence Who watches over every one of His creatures. Here are the concluding lines:

"To Him I entrust my spirit,
When I sleep and when I wake.
As long as my soul is with my body,
The Lord is with me; I am not afraid."

"Please Be With Us – My Husband is Dying"

When I arrived at my office in the morning, the voice mail had a message: "Please be with us. My husband is dying." I rushed to their room, where the nurse uttered a sigh of relief at my coming. The patient, who had been in our hospital for three months, was now expiring. I recited the proper prayers in the presence of his wife and teenage stepson.

After an hour in the room and with his mother in the hall, the stepson, a yeshiva student who had kept calm on the outside, suddenly felt faint and started collapsing. I managed to catch him under his arms, call for help, and have him taken to the TV room, where the nurse revived him with some fluids. The patient died later that morning, and I assisted the family in making plans for the removal of the body.

The nurse of Guggenheim 3 became so attached to this family that on the next day, her day off, she attended the funeral and chauffeured the family to the cemetery and back in her car – an act of great compassion indeed. I nominated her for a Service Award.

Establishing Priorities – One Problem at a Time

He was in a car accident which necessitated leg surgery. During the operation, cancer was discovered in that leg, and he had to stay in our hospital for a long time. He was beset by many problems, which just overwhelmed him. In my counseling, I suggested he list the problems in order of their priority, and handle one problem at a time. We worked out such a schedule, and his problems became manageable. Yet he was still depressed and requested that we pray together, after which he asked for a Bible in English translation. I provided him with one in modern English, as well as a book in contemporary Jewish personalities for lighter reading. He was highly appreciative of my efforts in his behalf.

Signing Surgical Consent Form

She was an elderly Holocaust survivor who needed open-heart surgery. Yet she was terribly frightened and refused to sign the consent form. Her daughter asked me to intervene. I talked to this patient in Yiddish, explaining why surgery was the only way to correct her problem and extend her life. On my recommendation, she signed the form, though hesitatingly. As promised, I visited her after surgery and continued to see her frequently, whenever she had her nurse call upon me.

The surgery was successful, though her later refusal to breathe for herself prolonged her stay at our CCU. After much soft talk to restore her will to recover and go home for the forthcoming Passover holiday, she rallied.

Presurgery Fright

This problem recurs very frequently and necessitates a great deal of emotional and spiritual support.

As I entered a private room, I found a complete family circle sitting around the patient silently and in a sullen, apprehensive mood. The patient, an elderly gentleman, was due for surgery that very morning. Tears came to his eyes. He was terribly frightened, and so was everyone else in the room. I was able to raise their spirits and strengthen confidence, hope, and reliance on Providence, in Whose hands all of us are. I prayed for the patient and gave him the text of a prayer he could recite himself before surgery. Then I told him that I planned to see him the following day and expected him, with God's help, to keep our appointment. He felt reassured. The morose atmosphere subsided. I did return the next day, and I visited him for several successive days afterward. He held my hand in his and expressed gratitude for my ministrations to him.

Reassuring a Cardiac Surgery Patient

At the conclusion of our hospital's Saturday services, the supervisor notified me that a patient in ACCU urgently requested my visit. I obliged, of course.

As I sat at his bedside, he related some of the highlights of his life. Then he spoke of his cardiac condition and the forthcoming surgery on Wednesday. What frightened him, he said, was that his surgeon had told him that one in 10,000 do not make it. I retorted that 9,999 do make it, and his chances are that he will be among the majority – easily. He felt somewhat reassured.

Then, on Monday night, Labor Day, the ACCU called me at home and said that the patient would undergo surgery on Tuesday morning and wanted to see me again right away. I went and found the patient tearful, frightened, beating his pillow, and so upset that the nurse could not determine his exact blood pressure. I let him have his cry but, as he persisted, I talked to him about the frequency of recovery from that surgery, about his being in the best possible condition for the next morning's surgery and about putting his life in God's Hands, trusting in God's mercy. I prayed for him in his room, and I told him I would do so again the next morning in my private worship. He appreciated it but requested that I see him again before surgery. I promised to do so, and added that I also planned to see him after surgery. In turn, I made a request of him: to remain calm and relaxed, and to try to get some sleep. He promised that and insisted on kissing my hand. I left him with his son at about 10:00 P.M.

When I visited him early next morning, I found him more relaxed and accepting the fact of surgery. I gave him reassurance and comfort. I then talked with his tearful wife in the hall and helped her regain her composure. Of course, I revisited this patient a number of times after surgery, called over a nurse to handle a problem, and left him relaxed and at ease.

Not Leaving a Worried Patient Alone

This patient had been transferred from CCU to a regular room a few days following heart bypass surgery. When I visited him, he asked me where he was and what had happened to him. Confusion had set in, yet he was fully aware of his forgetfulness. Concerned about his health, I approached his staff nurse and requested that the patient's physician be apprized of his condition. "I just don't feel right about leaving," I told her.

After a resident tested the patient, both he and I talked to the patient's physician on the phone and urged him to come. An elevated level of blood sugar had caused the forgetfulness and confusion. The patient was given insulin, and the physician ordered testing the patient's blood sugar regularly four times a day.

Reserving a Grave

This Russian-Jewish hospital employee had no family in this country, but he wanted to make sure that at the end of his earthly pilgrimage, he is buried in a Jewish cemetery. He turned to me for help. I located a respectable Jewish burial society that sells graves. It turned out that they offered two options: a reasonable membership fee plus yearly membership dues or one lump sum with the provision of paying it off in monthly installments. Since this employee had a heart condition, only the second option was available to him. I intervened with the society, then explained its offer to our employee. Then I steered him away from a cemetery where, in my rabbinic practice, I had frequently found the ground waterlogged to one where the ground is dry and the upkeep is good.

Touching the Blind

From time to time, one finds an inscription at the head of a bed noting that the patient is blind. This information is very helpful to the visiting chaplain since, without it, one would often not guess that the open eyes of the patient do not see. In such situations, I take the patient's hand into mine to replace eye contact during our conversation.

From a Former Patient

Thank you so much for your wonderful presence in my life. I truly appreciate it, my dear, dear Rabbi.

Finally Able to Cry

As I led the Sabbath morning service, I was surprised to see one woman sit and cry. Since it was a controlled cry and did not interrupt our worship, I decided to wait till after the service to have a chat with that patient. How surprised was I, therefore, when she came over to me during the *Kiddush*, of which she partook, and offered thanks for finally having been able to have a cry – something she was not able to do despite the great need she felt for relief through tears. A more relaxed and composed patient emerged from that Saturday service.

Israeli Knesseth Member at His Mother's Bedside

A key leader in the Israeli government coalition, a member of the Knesset (Parliament) and an ordained rabbi, came to our hospital to be at his mother's bedside in Falk ICU. I invited him and his sister to be my guests for the Sabbath. Though the president of The Mount Sinai Hospital had graciously placed a bed in his office for this most respected visitor, the rabbi felt he would be more comfortable in my home, where the Sabbath is observed in a traditional manner. The love and devotion he and his sister and the family displayed to a terminally ill mother were most touching to observe. What was also very moving were the words of good-bye and wishes for long life that the mother uttered to her adult children, after which she gave a kiss to each. The terminal stage lasted a week, during which she fell into a coma. The Israeli leader and I then said the Confession at her bedside. I also saw her and the devoted family circle daily and, at times, twice daily, and I offered comfort and support. I must single out our nursing staff at Falk's for the sympathy and understanding they showed to this closely knit family circle that so poignantly felt the suffering and coming loss of an aged mother.

Swallowing Pills

This gentleman, a cardiac patient, could not adjust to the hospital regimen and nervously kept on swallowing nitroglycerin pills. He complained to me about this habit of his. I was trying to relax him, and he turned the conversation to a great rabbinic authority of whom, he proudly stated, he was the fifteenth generation descendant. He regretted not having received any significant Jewish background. He had a book in English about his ancestor that meant very much to him. I left him in good spirits after mentioning that God bestows the merits of one's ancestors on their descendants and will mercifully grant him recovery.

$50,000 – for a Pill!

I spent a full hour listening to this patient, a Holocaust survivor who had done well in this country. He had given his children advanced religious and general education but felt hurt by one of his children. Then, turning the conversation to his illness, which he knew was very serious, he suddenly blurted out: "I do not want to suffer these pains from my illness. I will give you $50,000. Have pity on me, and get me a pill to end my life."

I was astounded to hear this but empathized with his sufferings. "My dear friend, *men tor nisht*," I told him in Yiddish. "That's strictly prohibited. Our hospital will do its very best for you. Remember, you are a religious man, and your family members died as martyrs. Remember who you are and what your heritage is." He calmed down somewhat, and I promised him future visits.

A College Freshman's Long Praying

A psychiatrist, knowledgeable in Judaism, asked me to have a talk with a patient: The young college freshman took very long to pray. He extended his praying, including the shortest Hebrew prayer, so long that his food got cold. I found the young man very sincere, talking about possibly studying for the rabbinate. He accepted my explanations of an I-Thou normal relationship and dialogue with God, in which exaggeration had no place.

Affection

A retired physician, a patient in our hospital, felt so uplifted by my visit that he took my hand, caressed his face with it, and kissed it. I was touched by this expression of affection.

"Help Me Again"

Message on my voice mail: "You helped me a lot before. Please help me again."

Russian-Jewish Child of Six

My attention was called to a six-year-old Russian-Jewish child who was born with a heart defect. Surgery was performed at Mount Sinai, and she was under constant treatment at the CCU. Then, fluids developed in her body, and surgery was again performed, this time to block a punctured lymph duct. I called my wife, who speaks Russian, and we stayed at the CCU till after 10:00 P.M. on a Saturday night and returned a few times the next day. The family kept vigil day and night. Unfortunately, the child passed on. But as the father of the child said, "The treatment here and in Russia is like day and night." Whatever was humanly possible to do was done here at our hospital.

Pathology Needed?

She had to undergo amputation of a leg. Her son requested that the leg be given to the family via a funeral director for burial, as Jewish law requires. However, after he signed the authorization, the secretary told him that pathology of the leg would be needed. That upset him. Upon consultation with his rabbi, he was told that it would be permissible only if the surgeon certifies that pathology of the severed limb was necessary to improve the mother's medical condition. The son, therefore, came to me, asking me to intervene and speak to the surgeon before the scheduled operation. It turned out that the surgeon had no need of the severed limb for pathology. I put the son on the phone to hear the surgeon's response, and he regained his peace of mind.

Deep Grief at Loss of Mother

I was urgently paged to see the daughter of a deceased patient in the day room of the floor. As I arrived, I heard the young woman's hysterical crying. Staff surrounded her, including the oncologist, social worker, and psychiatrist, but she was inconsolable. She had witnessed the death of her mother to whom, she kept on emphasizing, she was strongly attached and whom she loved deeply. She was an only child and kept accusing herself of not having done enough to save her mother's life. She enumerated a list of possible deeds she had missed, and those deeds, she claimed, might have been of medical benefit to her mother. With tears flowing from her eyes, she actually shouted her grief and her guilt of omission.

I took her hand and tried to tell her that it is very common and very human for family to feel that more could have been done, but that everything that could have been done was literally done. The social worker too tried to offer her some relief. Yet she said that she should have died instead of her good and beloved mother. As she kept repeating accusations against herself, we then witnessed the oncologist detail the medical efforts made for her mother. He added that her suggestions, insofar as they had some validity, had been tried. He must have talked to her for at least a full hour, responding to her every point. We all admired this good physician for the time he contributed and, of course, for his attempt to give her peace of mind. After a two-hour session, this loving bereaved daughter calmed down. "You were a blessing to your mother," I said to her as we parted.

"You really think so, Rabbi?" she asked.

"I am sure of that," was my response. I gave them information about preparations for the funeral service, and so, together with her father who had arrived and the social worker, she proceeded to make the necessary telephone calls to her rabbi and funeral parlor.

Cry to Dying Patient: "Don't Leave Me"

An emergency call on my beeper brought me to the room of this dying patient. The husband, in particular, was devastated and cried to his dying wife, "Don't leave me." The nurse tried very hard to calm him down. As I recited the Last Confession in Hebrew and English, he recognized the sentence of the *Shema* ("Hear, O Israel, the Lord is our God, the Lord is one,") and repeated it in the highest pitch of his voice in Hebrew. His daughters requested the prayer text and recited it themselves. The family was visibly and uncontrollably shaken.

Following this outburst of pain and grief, the husband mentioned that he had recently donated a Scroll of the Torah to his synagogue and would appreciate having his rabbi present at the hospital. That rabbi would also perform the funeral. I obliged and called the rabbi, urging him to come by taxi. In the meantime, I recited prayers aloud, mostly Psalms in Hebrew, at the bedside of the dying patient, and this had the additional effect of calming and keeping a mood of reverence and self-control in the room. Subsequently, I recited the prayer for the dying.

Physician Asks About Cremation

A physician, a member of our staff, called about a rather unusual problem. A patient of his died at another hospital and left a request in his will that his body be cremated. This upset the family, and the physician turned to me for guidance. I told him that, in a low-key fashion, he should explain the following to the family:

Jewish tradition considers the body as the handiwork of God and the temple of the soul. When a person dies, the body must be treated respectfully and returned to the earth where a natural decomposition takes place. We are not allowed to place the body into a fire and burn it. All of us have read about the crematoria in which the Nazis burned so many of our people. We do not want to do the same to someone we love, indeed to anyone. Moreover, Jewish religious law clearly rules that such a request in a will must not be carried out. In fact, one would be in violation of Jewish law if one carried it out. This is similar to one requesting his survivors do an illegal act which, of course, no one would carry out. The physician was truly gladdened to hear what Judaism teaches and thanked me, adding, "I am so glad I talked to you."

"I Have No Fear of Death"

She was a Holocaust survivor who had settled in Latin America. Yet, she related to me, her husband gave up everything in order to move to the United States, where he felt it was easier to raise children to be completely religious. Now, with the husband gone, and she being a patient at our hospital, she greeted me cheerfully. She proudly stated that though she was close to four-score years, she had no fear of death. She added, while raising her hands to heaven, "When I feel that my time is up, I will express hearty thanks to God for having enabled me to leave children, grandchildren, and even a great-grandchild in this world. All of them are religious *'zu Gott und zu leit'* – relating well and fully to God and fellow man. I am at peace with God. I will be leaving generations of good Jews." I wished that lady good health and many more years of life. While she extended appreciation and blessings to me for my visit, I kept thinking of the true success of her life and the happiness she feels in being continued spiritually by the next generations.

12: GUILT

How to Make Up with Offended Friends

A young religious collegian and psychiatric patient was perturbed because he felt he had offended his friends, and he asked how to make amends. We advised him to approach them before the Jewish High Holy Days and tell them the following: "Soon, we are going to ask God's forgiveness on Yom Kippur. Before I do that, I wanted to ask your forgiveness for any deed or verbal expression by which I may have offended you. Of course, I also forgive you for anything you may have done or said which could be offensive to me."

After listening to my advice, the young patient felt a sense of relief, for I had offered him a respectful way to make up which did not affect his self-esteem and, at the same time, was in harmony with Jewish religious practice during the holy season.

"Don't Respond"

A married daughter spent a month's time day and night in the private room of her ailing mother at our hospital. Yet the mother constantly criticized her son-in-law and disparaged her daughter's marriage, although she had found hospitality in their home. My advice to the devoted daughter was not to respond at all to her mother's invectives. In this case, silence seemed to me to be the best means of avoiding arguments and upsetting the patient by contradicting her. It should be sufficient compensation for the daughter to know that before God and man she is a caring daughter.

"I Wish I Could Make Up"

This patient, very gifted and successful in his profession, became dangerously ill and checked into our hospital, which did its utmost for him. He understood his condition and wanted me at his bedside very often. On one side, he expressed his pride in being a Jew. On the other side, he kept on repeating that he was a bad man and wished he could make up for it. Unfortunately, it was no longer possible "to make up." And so, as he held my hand in his and often kissed it, I encouraged him to think of the good deeds he had done in his life. Often, I just stood by his bedside, holding hands and listening as he tried to unburden himself of what weighed on his mind. During those times when we were together and I offered him words of comfort, he felt calm and serene. Incurably ill, the Lord spared him prolonged suffering.

A Measure of Comfort to Dying and Living

Her husband met me on a KCC floor and asked me to visit his wife, who, he said was dying. She was a middle-aged woman, fully conscious, and she raised the issue of God's reward to her for having meticulously carried out the laws governing Jewish family life. "The reward for the righteous," I told her, quoting the sages, "is mainly in the World to Come. However, the good you have done is well recorded in the heavenly books. And just as children can draw on their parents' bank deposits financially, so will your children benefit from the deposit of good deeds you have made in God's bank. '*Veoseh hesed laalofim*,' says the Torah in the second Commandment (Exodus 20:6), God 'shows mercy for generations of those who love Him and keep His commandments.' In the future your children and their families will benefit from your spiritual deposits now."

The dying patient found a measure of comfort in my reply. Her husband addressed the two daughters who sat at the bedside: "Remember what the rabbi has said," adding a measure of comfort to the children as well.

Guilt About Refusal to Change Burial Place

She had a nurse call me up for an urgent visit. Problem: She and her husband had reserved side-by-side plots in a cemetery. Her husband took ill, and a month before his death, he suddenly asked that he be buried next to his mother – who was in a different cemetery. They had had a good and long marriage, and she was surprised by this request. After his death, she and her children decided to bury him in the original plot. Then, a month after the funeral, she got sick and had to be hospitalized. This frightened her, as she attributed her illness to a kind of curse for not having fulfilled her husband's last wish. Now she was tearful, depressed, and felt guilty. She turned to me for guidance and relief.

In our conversation, it became clear that this couple loved each other and planned to be together after death as well – as proved by the purchase of joint graves. It also became clear that his relationship with his mother had not been a good one. Why then did he want to be buried near her? It was, I suggested, a seeking of protection in time of crisis – a kind of regression to childhood when one runs to Mother after getting hurt. Moreover, there were no empty graves near his mother, which meant he would have to be buried some distance away from her anyway. So why not be buried next to his wife in a different cemetery since it was impossible for her too to be buried near his mother? And, of course, the Jewish religion only allows exhumation in very rare cases, and this was not one of them.

This explanation registered with our patient. She was particularly grateful to hear me say that her husband had loved her until the end of his life, and his request to be near his mother was a relapse into childhood behavior. I left this patient relaxed and unburdened of a heavy yoke. I have seen her since then on regular visits and found her at peace with herself.

Relieving Tension

He was a very religious man who planned on taking over an institution for young people in Jerusalem. He had undergone bypass surgery in our hospital, and now felt tense and frightened after overhearing his two physicians talking about a transfer to another unit and more surgery. He was almost in tears about his condition. The nurses referred me to the resident on that floor, who, at my suggestion and in my presence, explained to the patient the treatment awaiting him. Yes, he would be transferred to our neurological unit. His arteries, which had clogged up, would be cleared and hooked up again. There was no danger involved, but it might take him two weeks to recover fully. Now, informed and relieved of his tension, he relaxed and spoke of his assignment in Israel.

Auto-Euthanasia?

She was a cancer patient who was still functioning relatively well. Her second husband, however, worried that he would eventually have to nurse her when her strength ebbs, and she is in pain and incapacitated. Therefore, he joined a society that advocated what they call "self-deliverance" or "auto-euthanasia" in cases of terminal illness. They describe methods to be used (drug doses) to accelerate the end in a legal way for the patient and the spouse. Our patient became terribly upset by her husband's plan to avoid taking care of her in such extreme circumstances. She rejected the plan for religious reasons as well, but did not know how to handle her husband. I advised her simply to tell him that there is another way out of his predicament: divorce. "Tell him," I suggested, "that you are ready to accept a divorce and in this way have him avoid all the hardship caused by a terminal wife. As for the financial settlement" – which had also entered the husband's considerations – "offer that he take two-thirds and you one-third of your common assets. This should make it more appealing to him."

Following our conversation, I am glad to say that the patient became more relaxed and regained her peace of mind. She had found an alternative to her dilemma. As her illness entered into remission, the husband did not press the issue.

Humor to Ease Malaise

On the general floors and in our ICU we often find patients who look uncomfortable with oral, nasal, and endotracheal tubes to which they are attached. Most of the time they cannot talk but their eyes tell you they appreciate your visit. After wishing them well and giving them a prayer text, I may add, "Please remember that those tubes are of benefit to you. They are also temporary. When you won't need them, they will be removed, and you will take your jacket, coat and umbrella and hitchhike home." This usually brings a smile to the patient's face or, if tubes block the mouth, smiling eyes plus a strong handshake. Tension and uncomfortable malaise are thereby reduced, and the patient gets to feel a little better about himself. Yes, humor, too, has a role in easing pressure.

Guilt Feelings

When the nurse saw me on her floor, she uttered a sigh of relief. She wanted me to have a chat with a troublesome, depressed patient who was difficult to handle. When I introduced myself, he immediately requested that we close the curtain. With tears in his eyes, he told me that he was making one step forward and two backward, and that God was getting even with him because he did not practice anything in Judaism, not even fasting on Yom Kippur.

I reassured him that God was forgiving; all he had to do was turn over a new page in the book of his life and promise himself that he would observe Yom Kippur and be a better husband from now on. I told him that God gives us new chances to improve ourselves and our relationship with Him. The next day, I brought him a booklet called *Faith in the Night*. His nurse assures me that she can handle him much better now and that he cooperates with her. In my weekly visits to him, he is much calmer and speaks of showing greater respect to his aged mother and to be a better husband and Jew.

Questions on Jewish Law

At times, I am called to see patients or their family members and answer their questions on Jewish law. A few examples:

- Maternity ward: What do you do when a boy is born circumcised? Answer: Only draw a drop of blood if no prepuce (foreskin) or mucous membrane as a sign of the covenant.

- Cremation problem: The wife of a terminal patient requested to see me. She told me of her plan to have her husband's body cremated and wanted to know my opinion on the subject. In a low-key fashion, I gave her reasons for not doing that. Her reaction: "You have convinced me, Rabbi. I will do as you suggest."
- Shivah (mourning): A patient told me that she had a very important question for me. She had been informed that her father had died. Her question: How can she observe shivah, the week of mourning, while at the hospital. I guided her in performing her shivah obligation in accordance with Jewish law and without having to leave her bed. I left her with peace of mind, Jewish law fulfilled, and hospital rules obeyed.
- Guidance of a student at KCC (Psychiatry) who wanted to become a Bible teacher.
- Lending prayer books to patients: So far, I have lent some of my personal books, and they were not returned. My reward will be if the patient recovers and uses my books frequently.

Recurrent Illness and its Tribulations

She was a very pious lady who covered her head with a kerchief, in the way of very religious Jewish women. She carried a heavy load on her mind. A constantly recurring infection, in addition to other medical problems, kept her in hospitals for long periods of time with no real cure in sight. Her preteen son now refused to speak to her because he felt his mother had abandoned him. The husband too had exhausted his patience. And there she was, alone with her thoughts and feelings in one of our rooms, seeing no solution to her troubles. Her faith had kept her going, and she still had enough of it to realize that the alternative – life without faith – had no meaning altogether. I listened to her litany of troubles and commiserated with her plaints to God for testing her so severely. I gave her the chance to unburden herself somewhat and tried to inject a note of hope. She knew that I prayed for her every Sabbath at the Torah and parted from me, saying, "Maybe your prayers for me will be answered." I felt humble before her suffering and, in leaving her, just said, "May God be merciful to you."

"What You Have Done for Me Is So Wonderful"

A social worker asked me to handle the case of a patient who was ridden with guilt. She had placed her aged mother in a nursing home and, two months later, her mother suddenly died at our hospital, where she had been taken for treatment, while the daughter, the present patient, was already hospitalized herself. I let the patient vent her feelings for a prolonged period of time while I remained a very attentive listener.

It turned out that her mother had raised her and her brother singlehandedly, having become an early divorcee. She had worked very hard, and her children had developed great attachment and admiration toward her. Later in life, our patient had taken her mother into her own home, and she had lived with her for nineteen years. However, when she herself became ill and unable to take care of her aged mother, her physician had insisted that she place her mother in a nursing home. A tremendous amount of guilt followed, and our social worker felt that only a rabbi could treat this patient.

I am glad to say that following my response, analysis, and discussion of her case, the patient regained her composure. We examined her total positive lifelong relationship with her mother and her medically confirmed inability to continue caring for the mother because of her own illness in the last two months of her mother's life. We concluded that she has, indeed, been an outstandingly supportive and loving daughter. The sudden death of her mother, I added, was a painless way of parting, something the Jewish tradition calls "the kiss of God."

Interestingly, ten days after our patient's discharge from our hospital, she called me up and said, "Something good happened inside me like a miracle. I keep thinking about all the things you told me, and I want you to know that what you have done for me is so wonderful." I then traced the Hebrew date of her mother's passing for her to keep the annual yahrzeit religiously. It happened to coincide with a Jewish holiday when the Yizkor Memorial Prayer is also recited, and so I advised her to go to the synagogue on that day particularly, and thereby be able to continue expressing her love and respect for her mother's memory.

13: BEREAVEMENT

Death of an Infant

My beeper went off on a Friday morning in wintertime. The clinical supervisor of the Pediatric ICU asked that I come up to her unit, where a six-month-old baby had died and the parents wanted to speak to me. I found a grieving mother sitting on a chair, a grandmother disconsolate, and a father talking on the phone while holding back his tears. I listened to their expressions of grief.

Then questions arose on funeral arrangements and on the applicability of Jewish religious law in that case. Usually, for an infant who has lived a month, mourning, shiva and kaddish are required. After speaking on the phone to the rabbi of the family's community and questioning the parents, the fact emerged that this baby had been on a respirator from the day following birth until now because it was not viable otherwise. In such a case, Jewish law rules that the child is in the category of a *nefel*, for whom regular burial is required but there is no shiva or kaddish. The family wanted to have the funeral that afternoon, but that became impossible because the cemetery personnel would leave at 1:30 P.M. Following the numerous calls the family asked me to make, it became clear that the funeral would have to be postponed till Sunday.

After being with the family for more than two hours and offering support, the initial shock subsided somewhat. I reminded the family that they were needed by the other children and turned their attention to raising them with love and attention. I also held out the possible prospect of another healthy child in the future. The nursing staff hugged the mother and grandmother good-bye, and the funeral director arrived and took the child's body. I recited Psalm 91 and then, at an intersection in the corridor, directed the family to their car while they expressed thanks to me for my help in their time of need.

Uproar in Emergency Ward

Someone had tried to beep me, but when I returned the call, nobody knew who needed me. So I continued handling problems in the Guggenheim

Building, where I was making rounds that afternoon. The patient representative stopped me and told me that the emergency ward was looking for me to handle a difficult case. A religious Jewish man had died, and staff and family were at a loss on how to proceed. A sigh of relief greeted me as I entered the office of the social worker, where everybody was assembled. It seemed they just could not agree on what funeral chapel to contact and were worried that the body would be taken to the morgue.

After offering sympathy to the bereaved wife of the deceased, I recommended that they take a funeral parlor in the neighborhood where they lived, so that neighbors and friends could come to the service and give honor to the deceased. After a brief conversation, I obtained a unanimous consent on one specific funeral parlor, which was immediately contacted. I gave the parlor some pertinent information and asked that they have the body removed without delay. They would obtain additional information from the family that evening, during a visit to their funeral chapel. A rabbi who was close to the family was also contacted and a message was left on his voice mail. All that was done in fifteen minutes, to the relief of all. The widow and staff were most grateful. Before leaving, I stressed that they give him a respectful funeral service, and that the deceased might most want to tell his wife to take good care of her health. "That's exactly what he told me this morning," she replied and shook my hand warmly.

Hospital Acts with Extra Compassion and Understanding to a Pious Family

The Hassidic patient had been in our hospital for weeks when the physicians briefed the family that he was terminal. The wife and daughter continued their vigil, tried to keep him comfortable, and recited Psalms. It was a Friday in the winter, and I was asked to help in resolving some special problems which arose. Indeed, this family's requests went beyond what a hospital is supposed to provide. Yet, because of the special circumstance of possible imminent death, the vice president of nursing permitted me to arrange the following:

Two people were allowed to stay in the patient's private room throughout the forthcoming Sabbath. Eight other children, including one who arrived from England, were to stay and sleep in a classroom on the same floor for the Sabbath. I arranged for our patient representative office to furnish the room with a few cots, and had a refrigerator brought in as well. During the death, the family wanted to be together in the patient's room. Should it occur on the Sabbath, the body was not to be removed to the morgue, and nurses were not to handle the body, but leave it for the Holy Society, which would come at the conclusion of the Sabbath. I left these written instructions for the floor's nursing supervisor and had the office state the same special arrangements in an official pass which was given to the family. "How can you take so much suffering by patients?" the daughter asked me. "By helping others and relieving the burdens they carry," I answered. The patient died on Saturday night past midnight in the presence of the whole family, thereby avoiding any religious problems. Our hospital had done more than duty and regulations require. The religious and emotional needs of this pious family were respected and fulfilled.

Help on a Sad Day

Dear Rabbi Spirn:

I would like to thank you for helping me on one of the saddest days of my life. The day my husband passed away. When I called on you at the Mount Sinai Hospital, you kindly helped my family and myself expedite the funeral arrangements for my husband.

Please accept my thanks for your kindness and caring.

Sincerely,

From Denial to Acceptance

Staff paged me to help calm a disconsolate woman, who was under shock at the passing of her mother. She cried bitterly and loudly and said she loved her mother and would take her home. She was totally unable to accept the fact that her mother was no longer alive. She just denied reality. Her brothers stood by her side and so did the floor's social worker – all trying to make her face reality. It took over an hour in that day room until, exhausted and in pain, she finally let go. While the social worker mentioned the hospital's need for the bed, which meant that the family's funeral director should be called soon to remove the body, I stressed the early coming of the Sabbath in the winter. I asked the daughter not to make her religious mother violate the sanctity of the day and call the funeral director at once. I praised the great devotion she had shown her mother, especially during hospitalization, and asked that mother now be given the rites prescribed by our religious tradition. Slowly, this grief-stricken mourner accepted the reality of the situation while I had her brothers call the funeral director before the early arrival of the Sabbath.

Losing a Sibling

Following our Saturday morning services, I went to see a few patients who needed some extra visiting when I suddenly heard loud crying from the consultation room of 10-Center. Almost immediately, a nurse noticed me and asked that I step into the room and extend help. An Iranian-Jewish patient whom I knew well had expired, and his siblings were crying hysterically and beating their bodies with their hands while sitting on the floor. (I suspected this was common practice in Iran and was not particularly worried about the bereaved.) Two nurses tried to calm them down by applying cold compresses dripping with water on the foreheads and faces of these mourners. However, the pain was too deep and the crying very acute. They were a religiously observant family and knew that such vociferous mourning was not permitted on the Jewish Sabbath, but they were just overwhelmed by their loss. We were also worried about upsetting the other patients on that floor. I spoke softly to them, words of consolation, and praised them for the constant care they had given their brother throughout his consuming illness. After two hours in that state, and after the deceased was moved to our morgue, a decision was reached to take them to the emergency room in wheelchairs for a medical check-up, after which they walked home.

Determining Time of Passing

The deceased had died in our hospital almost a year ago. Now the family was ordering a tombstone, and they were unsure if he had passed away before or after sunset – which would affect the date on the Jewish calendar. The Young Israel organization to which they had turned advised them to contact me. I immediately called our supervisor of medical records, and within half an hour he found the answer. Death had occurred well past sunset, so that the Hebrew date would have to be the date of the next day. When I called the deceased's brother with the information, he broke out in tears, again feeling the pain of his loss. I calmed him with words of solace, finishing our brief conversation in a way that enabled him to regain his composure.

"Nothing Remained of My Mother"

She was a patient in our psychiatric ward. Following Sabbath services, she spoke to me about herself, her career as a writer, and her grief at having lost her mother recently. She also requested that I visit her. When I did, she was very nervous and asked that I hold her hand. She told me that she was returning home the next day and felt apprehensive about it. Upon further inquiry, it appeared that her psychiatrist approved of her leaving and that she would continue her medication at home under the supervision of private nurses, whom her family could afford. Preparing to go home reminded her of her mother's absence. She had felt very close to her and asked that we offer a prayer for her deceased mother. During the short prayer she burst out crying and said, "Nothing remained of my mother. She was cremated and my father keeps her ashes in a closet." I offered some possible comfort, adding that the soul is not perishable and so she can still pray for her mother's soul. I then elaborated on her returning to familiar surroundings and to a profession in which she feels a sense of fulfillment, and in which she will find recognition through publishing. As I described her future, the anxiety of leaving the hospital subsided, and a smile appeared on her face. "I may call on you to perform my wedding," she said in parting, with a big smile on her face. "With a Jewish boy," I replied, and she repeated my words with a smile.

Tears for Having Missed His Father's Yahrzeit

We conversed for a while, and as happens so often in my chaplaincy, he felt a closeness to me and asked for my help with a problem that weighed heavily on his mind. With tears in his eyes, he related that he had to be rushed to our hospital on the very anniversary of his father's passing and, therefore, for the first time in his life he missed observing the yahrzeit because he was unable to attend religious services and recite kaddish. As he talked, I noticed the scars of heart bypass surgery on his chest. I answered him feelingly that his omission was not voluntary but clearly and urgently needed by his cardiac problem. Jewish tradition does not obligate a person to do what is truly impossible for one to do. Moreover, our tradition obligates one to seek immediate help in case of danger. This explanation offered him only some comfort, and so it dawned on me that if I could offer him a way of making up for his omission, he would regain his peace of mind. Since the next Yizkor memorial service was going to be on Yom Kippur, I suggested that after reciting the Yizkor prayer in memory of his father, he also recite the *Molay Rachamim* prayer ("O God, full of mercy..."), which is usually offered at a yahrzeit. And, of course, he may recite kaddish on that holiest of days. This religious prescription of mine accomplished wonders: It is religiously valid and emotionally proved to be a full remedy to this sensitive man's feeling of guilt. I left him a man at peace with himself.

Checking Himself Out?

This man had been a very difficult patient in our psychiatric ward. He also requested frequent sessions with me, during which he vented all his grievances against staff.

High-strung as he was, he had decided to check himself out of our hospital. His psychiatrist then requested that I try to persuade him to withdraw his seventy-two-hour notice of leaving, as he was absolutely not ready to go home. I am glad to state that the patient, who called me "his rabbi," did withdraw his notice in writing, to the full satisfaction of the physician.

Departed with Dignity and Respect, Thanks to You

Dear Rabbi Spirn,

Your kind expression of sympathy is gratefully acknowledged and deeply appreciated.

The family wishes to thank you very much for all that you did for us in our time of need. Your words and actions were a comfort to us all. Thanks to you, she received all the dignity and respect that she deserved.

Dilemma About Lonesome Patient

One of our medical students called me up to tell me that, while he was shopping at a supermarket, he saw an elderly lady collapse. He immediately dialed 911-emergency, and the lady was taken to our hospital. He asked me to follow up this case, since he found out that she was Jewish. It turned out that she was put on a respirator and, soon afterward, was declared brain dead. Nobody knew if she had any relatives. Following one clue, I called the office of one of our physicians, whose patient she had been, and received her home address but nothing more. We then felt that perhaps one of her neighborhood synagogues might know the name of a relative or a friend of hers. I called five synagogues plus Hadassah, of which she was a member, but no additional information was available. Taking precautions, I had our nursing staff put the following information into her chart:

1.As the head chaplain of the hospital, I oppose an autopsy on religious grounds.

2.If no relative is found, contact the Hebrew Free Burial Association.

I also suggested that our legal department obtain permission to search her apartment for names of relatives, or to go over and speak to the superintendent of her building. That, indeed, provided the solution. The superintendent had the telephone number of a nephew who lived in a different state. The nephew was notified and came to the Mount Sinai. I considered my task finished only when I met the nephew, and he took over all the arrangements for the funeral.

"Blessed Be the True Judge"

When I knock at a patient's door and get no answer, I open it slightly and ask in a loud voice if I may enter. Most of the time, the room is empty, as the patient must have gone for treatment. In such cases, I leave my visiting card, which has my name and phone number. However, occasionally, with a sudden shock, I see a sheet-wrapped and strapped body in a supine position in the center of the bed or an immobile body covered to the neck with a bed sheet, with eyes closed and mouth open. The patient had died, and our staff had proceeded to the postmortem care done for all deceased patients except the Orthodox and Hassidic Jews, who are handled by the Holy Society (*Chevrah Kadisha*). Finding such a body, I can only offer a Psalm and the prayer "Blessed be the true Judge" – expressing our submission to the Divine decree.

2:30 A.M. to 5:30 A.M. at the Hospital

September 10, 1992

Dear Rabbi Spirn:

I am writing upon the conclusion of shiva for my brother to thank you on behalf of our family for your kindness and assistance.

When I called you at the time of my brother's admission to Mount Sinai Hospital, you immediately sprang into action. Your visits were comforting to him and it was reassuring to know that you were available and eager to be of service.

When my brother passed away unexpectedly at 2:00 A.M. only four days later, and we requested that you be paged, you responded quickly and were immensely helpful to us at that tragic time. Although our loss was enormous, you made it easier for my sister-in-law and other members of the family who were present to do what had to be done. We will always be grateful to you.

May Hashem [God] reward you with *nachas* [happiness] from your family and good health and strength to continue your vital work.

Mount Sinai Hospital is fortunate to have a chaplain with your ability, sincerity and dedication.

Sincerely yours,
Rabbi ---

Transporting a Deceased on the Sabbath?

She died on a Friday afternoon in the winter – a time when the Sabbath begins at about 4:00 P.M. Her mother consulted me on how to proceed, as she had contacted a funeral parlor from upstate New York, where the family resides. My advice: let that upstate Jewish funeral director have a New York City director pick up the body and keep it during the Sabbath. Then, on Saturday night, after the conclusion of the Sabbath, the body can be moved upstate. This way, one avoids traveling with a Jewish deceased on the holy Sabbath day. The mother and the funeral director accepted my recommendation.

"I Want My Dad"

As I was about to leave the hospital in the evening, the telephone rang, and a nurse in S-4 asked for help. It involved a middle-aged woman who could not handle her grief at the demise of her father. She kept on talking to and kissing her father, asking God and him why he left her. She had never married but remained a homemaker, taking care of her father, to whom she showed extreme devotion. He was also her only interest in life. "I want my dad," she kept crying. At one point she said she noticed movement of the bedsheet with which her father was covered and insisted that he was still breathing. I asked for the physician's complete reexamination of the deceased. The physician carefully checked both the breathing and the circulation and reassured the daughter that her father was not alive. The daughter calmed down somewhat. Yet, as she was unable to make decisions, I called her cousin, and we made arrangements with a funeral chapel to remove the body from the hospital. Before leaving, I also counseled the daughter in ways to overcome her loneliness and her feeling of abandonment. I spent two hours on this case and was grateful for having been able to help this family in a trying time.

Shock of Sudden Death – Body to Hungary

Staff of our Falk ICU called to ask for my immediate intervention with a lady who had just found out that her husband had expired. I found her crying in the unit's waiting room and constantly asking why her gravely ill husband had been moved from FICU to the Medical Special Care Unit, where he had died upon arrival. She had no children and no family in this city, and her husband's nurse called the woman's friends to come over promptly.

I reconstructed the day's happening: Her husband was supposed to go to our MSCU in the first place. However, because of lack of a free bed, he was taken to the FICU. That morning, though, the physician of the MSCU had seen the patient and decided to have him transferred to the MSCU. This was explained to the patient's wife but she remained inconsolable.

At her request, I contacted the night administrator, asking that the body remain in the MSCU till the wife's friend arrived, so that both might see him a last time and bid farewell. We also requested that the body remain in the morgue through the night as the wife wished to call the Hungarian consulate in the morning, to obtain permission to transfer the body for burial among his family members in Hungary. The administrator approved both requests.

Following the arrival of a friend, I expressed sympathy to the bereaved, lonely wife, urged her to watch over her own health and commended her for the devotion she had shown her husband throughout his illness. His physician met me in the hall a few days later and expressed his gratitude to me for the manner in which I handled this bereaved wife. He also told me that she had succeeded in transferring her husband's body for burial in Hungary.

Supporting a Bereaved Family – Body to Brazil

They were a Syrian-Jewish family who had settled in Brazil. One of them, a young married man in his thirties, was brought over to our Medical Special Care Unit in KCC 3 following a stroke. His pregnant wife, father-in-law, and brother had all come over as the patient went into a coma. A few days later he died. Conversing with the family in French, I assisted them in making all arrangements for the transportation of the body to Brazil. At the same time we offered a degree of spiritual support, especially to the young pregnant widow, who seemed inconsolable.

Lone Professor's Remains Sent to Niece in Israel

He was an Israeli professor who was teaching in American colleges. He spent a few weeks as a patient in our hospital, and I visited him frequently. Then, on a Sunday afternoon, the hospital called me at my home to tell me that he had died that morning. Since he had no relatives in this country, I was given the phone number of his niece in Israel, and, furthermore, I was asked to have an Orthodox funeral director prepare the body for burial and send it to Israel.

This required someone who not only knew his profession and was Orthodox but could also obtain the necessary authorizations from the Consulate of Israel in New York City and would accept payment by the niece living in Israel. We established a three-way telephone conversation with Israel, getting all the information we needed. As the niece's son unexpectedly came to this country, our director of security had the professor's belongings given to me to assume responsibility, and I passed them on to the niece's son.

Our hospital staff was much relieved to have me handle this difficult situation.

Italian-Jewish Body Sent to Italy

A nurse called me from the FICU about a terminal patient whose family, now residents of this country but not of New York City, wanted to fulfill his wish to be buried in Italy, near the graves of his dear ones. I saw this family a number of times. I guided them, providing the information needed to fulfill the patient's wish. When he passed on in Oncology, where he had been moved, a nurse called on me to pronounce the proper prayers and also to be with his wife and children during that sorrowful, painful time.

Soliloquy on Religion Before Dying

He had me paged. As I sat in his room, he spoke about the importance of religion. His condition was poor, and I spent much time listening to his elaborate soliloquy. Of course, I offered some comfort to him. Then, the next day, he died.

The supervising nurse of his floor contacted me about the removal of his body, which had remained untouched in his room as he was listed as an Orthodox Jew. Six hours after the family had been notified of his passing, no one had arrived. Since the patient was unmarried, I contacted his brother and he, after giving all the pertinent information to his rabbi, had the local funeral director contact me.

Apparently there was a misunderstanding between the funeral director and our staff. The director had wanted to be contacted when the death certificate was ready. This was not understood by the staff, so each one waited for the call of the other party. After putting all concerned in touch with each other, we resolved the problem and the body was released seven to eight hours after death had occurred. May Heaven accept the soul of this suffering patient whose last conversation was a soliloquy on the importance of religion.

An Unexpected Request

She was an elderly lady. After I introduced myself, she immediately asked me to find a place for her in a cemetery. Upon inquiry, she revealed she had no plot reserved anywhere and, having no family, she wanted to be certain she would be buried in a Jewish cemetery. She belonged to no synagogue and no organization, she said, and therefore I was the only one to turn to for help. Looking for some clue, I questioned her about her husband, and that gave me a solution. She named the cemetery in which her husband was buried, and remembered the name of the synagogue to which that ground belonged and the year of her husband's passing. With that information at hand, I made the proper contacts and helped this patient.

Judge in a Coma

This American Jewish judge came to us as a very sick man after having been in other hospitals. He went into a coma three days after his arrival. His wife spent every day at his bedside for more than half a year. Although not formally religious, the wife had strong spiritual values. When he developed high fever and other complications and the physician suggested letting him die in peace, his wife turned to me for a decision based on Judaism on whether to let the doctor refrain from giving her husband elaborate life support treatment, thus letting him die. Judaism rules that one must continue to help the patient. She abided by it. I also told her that following our religious teachings will also give her inner satisfaction that she had refused to shorten her husband's life.

She regularly attended our Sabbath services for inspiration and strength and for the opportunity to be present at the Torah when I offered a prayer for her husband's well-being. During one false weekday alarm about imminent death, she called, and I immediately went to see her and be at her side.

In a letter to our hospital, which the director forwarded to me, she wrote: "I intend to continue to attend services as long as my husband is in the hospital. I hope Rabbi Spirn will continue to help us all in our time of sorrow. His sermons are very inspirational and uplifting. His sermons are very moving. He has given me spiritual assistance in this trying time. His visits to me at the hospital have brought me much solace."

In a note to me, the director added: "I thought you would like to see how much your spiritual guidance is appreciated in times of sorrow."

No Chapel Service?

The family of an expired patient wanted to avoid a chapel service. I advised that the funeral parlor prepare the body for Jewish burial and that a graveside service be held in the presence of their rabbi.

Israeli Comatose Patient

I received a call from out-of-town to please counsel the family of a comatose patient at our hospital, an Israeli. As I reached his floor, I found his aged mother, his sisters, and his niece outside his room, all on edge. They had come from Israel and were all perturbed by what they considered insufficient care by the physicians.

I called the patient's physician, and he claimed that the problem was the family's refusal to accept the fact of approaching death. He said he had forty patients in his waiting room but would come nonetheless if there was any hope. I explained to him that, in Jewish tradition, as long as there is life we must preserve it and try to prolong it. In response, despite his pessimism, the physician obliged and came to the room. In the meantime, I traced the oncology specialist who had promised the family to come, and he too obliged and came right away. Both physicians then reexamined the patient and agreed on a course of action. The family was so grateful!

A Synopsis of the Laws of Mourning at an ICU

His father was on the critical list in our Falk ICU. He asked many questions related to his father's possible death just before or during Rosh Hashanah, as well as detailed questions on the observance of shivah (seven days of mourning) and the year of mourning. He insisted on writing down my replies so as to ensure his proper observance. He had established a very friendly rapport with the rabbi of the Lubavitch synagogue in the Far West, where he had settled, and so I offered to give him the phone number of the Lubavitch headquarters in Brooklyn, where he could ask for the rabbi's prayers on his father's behalf. I also recited the Confession (*Viduy*) at his father's bedside and gave him the text of the prayer for the dying, to be recited when staff notices the ebbing of life. Two days later, on the morning before Rosh Hashanah, the father expired. I offered sympathy and guided the family in their decision to hold the funeral after the holiday.

Minyan in Semiprivate Room at Time of Expiration?

One of our nurses called for my help with a serious problem. A group of ten Hassidic students, constituting a quorum called a minyan, insisted on being at the bedside of a dying patient, while the roommate strenuously objected to having such a crowd in their small room. After much discussion, the two sons of the terminal patient were allowed to stay near their mother, as it is a religious duty to stand by the dying person and offer prayers when death is about to occur. The rest of the Hassidim, however, understood the problem and left gracefully.

Unjustified Fear of Death

On a Sunday night, I was contacted about an unruly man in one of our ICUs. I came over immediately and noticed that three nurses were on duty in the unit, even though this patient was the only one there. He felt he was going to die that night and was continuously alarming the nurses. Medically, however, there was no cause for alarm. The rhythm of his heart (his medical problem) was well under control through drugs, and the nurses were monitoring it carefully. I spent an hour with this patient, reassured him and told him that his prognosis was good and that, with God's help, he had many years of life ahead of him. He kept asking me to spend the whole night at his bedside. I told him I would not do it because I was confident that nothing would happen to him. Then, I prayed aloud for him and left him with a promise that I would see him again very soon. On my next visit, he looked relaxed and told me he had apologized to the nurses for the hard time he had given them that Sunday night. The nurses confirmed this. I am glad to state that the patient recuperated beautifully and was "honorably discharged."

There is a Limit to Reciting the Mourner's Kaddish

After a conversation I handed her a prayer card, as I do to most patients. She asked if it contained the kaddish. It turned out that she had the habit of reciting that prayer for the deceased every day for a decade, in memory of her long-gone parents. Whereupon I remarked that kaddish is recited only during eleven months after the passing of a parent, and later only on yahrzeit – the anniversary of the passing of a close relative. We also recite the Yizkor memorial prayer four times a year on Jewish festivals, thereby keeping the memory of a loved one alive and sacred; all that but no more. Judaism wants us to turn away from becoming morose. It guides us toward facing life and its requirements. By living a virtuous, good life, we automatically add merit to our deceased parents. She listened carefully, and, I trust, will redirect her thoughts toward life.

Guiding a Friend of a Deceased Patient

She was a terminal patient with no family, and had only a friend who was named the executrix of her will. On the physician's recommendation, the friend contacted me and asked for my help. She had no knowledge of what to do when the patient passes away. After discussing all the details, I offered to insert a request into the patient's chart that, upon her expiration, I should be notified day or night by our hospital's staff. I received such a call at 6:30 A.M. the next morning and then notified the executrix of the will, who, at that point, knew how to proceed.

Too Poor to Buy a Burial Place

The Russian-Jewish family had been in this country only five years. Unfortunately, the father had died on the operating table. It was not cardiac surgery, but his heart just stopped. Now they were all forlorn, not knowing what to do next, and I was called to offer help. Since they were rather poor, I referred them to the Hebrew Free Burial Association, which gave them the help needed. No question of autopsy was raised, and that gave the family some peace of mind.

Rabbit on Grave

He was a Yiddish poet coming back to our hospital for another stay. His family called me up, and I went to see him immediately. The next day, on the Sabbath, I spent an hour with him, and he said the visit gave him much comfort. Then, on Monday, he called and requested another immediate visit.

He had written a poem in Yiddish and had had it translated into English by a friend of his. However, the translator had mistakenly translated the title of the poem "The Little Donkey" instead of "The Little Rabbit." The patient wanted me to have the page-and-a-half poem retyped, inserting the word "rabbit" wherever it said "donkey." The poem, which was very moving, was dedicated to his late wife, whose grave he had visited and had discovered that a little rabbit had made its home on the grave. This poet found it very meaningful that, out of all the graves, the rabbit had somehow chosen the one of his dear wife. For after the Holocaust, had not his wife brought aid and consolation to many Jewish orphans who had remained all alone after the war? Now this little rabbit too had found a place of rest near this protective Jewish mother. Of course, I had the poem retyped promptly and returned it to him for publication.

Renewed Appreciation – Eleven Years Later

September 5, 1994

Your kind expression of sympathy was deeply appreciated and is gratefully acknowledged by the family of ---

Dear Rabbi Spirn:

It was so good to hear from you once again, despite the fact that your warm and caring note arrived at this sad time in my life. Your words brought much comfort to me, as did your presence more than eleven years ago when we first met at the Mount Sinai Hospital when my husband was hospitalized for nine weeks. Those were terrible times, too, but your presence then was a source of strength and helped to sustain us. Now, too, may God bless you and your lovely family with much *nachas* for the new year and always, and may He give you health and strength to continue to do your good work for many years to come. I am sending a small contribution to whatever good work it can best serve.

Fondly,

To Tell or Not to Tell a Teenager?

They had thought he was sleeping so long as a result of a pill given to him, but soon his physician concluded that the patient was in a coma. His wife, therefore, asked me to offer the proper rites. I obliged and recited the Confession (*Viduy*) and then the prayer for the dying. For a long time I remained with the wife and a college-age daughter, both of whom shed tears, grieving over the anticipated loss. Then the question arose on whether to allow a teenage daughter to come to the hospital in order to fulfill her wish to see her father once more. Following a private conversation with the patient's oncologist, whom I noticed in the hall, I advised the family to disclose any shocking information to the teenager only when one of them is with her, not by phone when she is home all alone. The procedure should be to first explain some positive aspects, namely that the father had had a full year of remission of his cancer through treatment and God's mercy. Now, too, he was in a coma and did not feel the pain in his liver, to which the cancer had gone by metastasis. These two points represented the silver lining of the tragedy. Then, I should be quoted as advising that it is best to remember the father the way he looked at last month's Passover Seder, which had been a happy one for the family. However, if she absolutely insisted on coming to the hospital, the family should not oppose the visit. The decision was hers, but she should keep the chaplain's advice in mind.

Terminal Patient Wants the Rabbi's Presence

In this case, the emaciated patient had called for me. Then, he asked for two skullcaps, one for him and one for his son. I sat at his bedside and in a low, soothing voice, recited prayers. The patient remained calm and peaceful. He rallied for a few days but the prognosis was tragically clear. His exhausted wife, who stayed for hours at his bedside every day, struggling to be as brave as possible, suddenly could not bear this suffering any longer. In the hospital hallway, she let her feelings go. I listened to her pain at such prolonged suffering with no chance of recovery. I also listened to her desperate espousal of euthanasia while counseling against it – as matters of life and death better remain in the hands of God above and not in the hands of humans who may abuse that right. I saw her at least five days in a row and offered a listening heart, understanding, and sympathy. Some time after her husband's death, she expressed her appreciation by sending a gift of $100 to our Jewish Chaplaincy Fund for the purchase of religious articles.

No Fees for Chaplain. Just Say Kaddish for Father

I had seen him during my regular visits. He came from Leningrad and had brought his complete family to New York. Then, on a late Sunday afternoon, the supervisor called me at my home to tell me he had died, and the family wanted to see me. I found his wife and four adult children in his room. They just did not know how to proceed with a funeral. Upon inquiry, it turned out that the deceased, who was a very religious man despite his upbringing under Communism, had joined a Washington Heights synagogue. It seemed logical, then, to have him buried in the congregation's cemetery plot. After numerous telephone calls to reach the rabbi and the funeral director and to obtain approval from the congregation, and after explaining funeral practices in this country, I resolved the problem. One of the deceased's sons, who told me he was employed professionally, then asked for my fees (!) for several hours of work. My reply was, "Say kaddish for eleven months in memory of your heroic father and relearn to put on the tefillin for prayer." I left after the body was removed, while the family and the supervising nurse expressed overwhelming gratitude to me.

Injection Needed to Calm Spouse

As I walked home from synagogue services one Saturday night, a hospital guard notified me that I was urgently needed at the morgue. There I found the night administrator, a physician, and two bereaved family members – the wife and son of a patient whom I had visited many times and whose heart had given way a few hours before. Their feelings were especially intense, since the patient had died most unexpectedly (he had been hospitalized for a different problem, not his heart condition). As the body was brought into the morgue, the son insisted on having his father's face uncovered and then, tearfully and hysterically, addressed his father. We just watched his display of grief and then slowly weaned him away from the dead man to assist his mother in making telephone calls to arrange the removal of the body to a funeral parlor. The mother had been given an injection to calm her down before my arrival.

The family did not have the name of a funeral home, nor did they have a cemetery plot. I guided mother and son, giving them not only information on how to proceed, but also soothing comfort. I calmed them down after answering their many religious questions.

Since rules require that anyone who received a calming injection be supervised for four hours and this family wanted to go home, the physician requested the signature of the deceased's wife, to release the hospital from responsibility. This was granted in my presence. However, at my suggestion, the physician gave the son the name of the medication administered and her own name and phone number to be used in case of aftereffects on the road home. I left them at 10:30 P.M. after the body was removed and the family drove home.

Shivah Observance at Hospital

Jewish law discourages divulging sad news to a patient for fear it will aggravate his condition. Still, the family and the physician felt that this man, who had undergone bypass surgery and was recuperating nicely, should be told that his beloved mother had died. Seven days of mourning (Shivah) followed. The patient insisted on saying kaddish at least during evening services. To offer him a measure of comfort, we made extra efforts to gather a quorum of ten men for minhah and maariv services.

Son of Physician in Oncology

His young bride was constantly at his bedside. Both said they regretted not having had a religious upbringing, which would have helped sustain them in those trying times. I offered comfort and solace for weeks. On the day of his passing, his wife could not be present for emotional reasons. His parents and a brother, however, were there. The father, a physician, took the son's pulse, stated that the end was near, and walked nervously in the room. I offered the prayer for the dying and, as I ended with the proclamation of the unity of God (the last words a Jew is to recite before death occurs), the young man expired. I stayed on till the family got involved in practical matters for removal of the body.

Suffering Spouse Unburdens Her Grief

It happened after the husband had been hospitalized for four months and was weakening. He was in the Neoplastic Division of our hospital, where I had visited him regularly and chatted with him. The agonized wife verbalized her struggle to save her husband's life. I listened carefully and feelingly. She spoke for an hour. Here was despair at man's utter helplessness – the last battle in which man is physically always the loser...

A Call for Help from California

A colleague of mine, chaplain at the Cedars-Sinai Hospital, called from Los Angeles to solicit our hospitality for his mother's neighbor in New York, whose husband was undergoing surgery at our hospital. The well-meant plea was really unnecessary in this case, because I had already invited this heartbroken lady to be my guest for the Sabbath. Both she and her husband were Holocaust survivors. As his stay became prolonged, either she or their son spent consecutive Sabbaths at my home.

The husband had his ups and downs and underwent emergency surgery just when he was on the verge of being discharged. Then our AICU paged me on my beeper. He had taken a sudden turn for the worse, and his heart gave way. I found the family in uncontrollable grief, and the surgeon explained to them, with warmth and compassion, that both surgeries had been successful when, unexpectedly, the heart stopped. It seemed to be a painful occurrence for the surgeon as well. For religious reasons, the family declined his request for an autopsy. I guided this grief-stricken family in their plans for burial in the Holy Land.

Months later, the widow called for words of comfort. All her children offered her love and a home – indeed, a blessing in modern times of broken family relationships. While crying on the phone, she listened to my heartfelt compassion for her and my emphasis that she must now act as both mother and, by proxy, father to such a loving family. She requested permission to call me up whenever needed, and I encouraged her to do so.

A Hassid's Mother's Death on the Sabbath

She had been a patient in our hospital a number of times when she expired on a Saturday morning. Her supervising nurse then came to see me in the auditorium where I led Jewish Sabbath services and asked for my visit to handle this case. I obliged at the conclusion of the services. The son of the deceased was a Lubavitcher Hassid and wanted to have his mother's body remain in the room until the evening, which marks the conclusion of the Sabbath. The usual practice is to move the body to the morgue unless it is close to the conclusion of the Sabbath. In this case, I pleaded with our staff to let the body remain in the private room for the remainder of the Sabbath day, as is recommended by Jewish law and out of respect to her religious feelings and to the son, who teaches at the Lubavitcher Yeshiva. Moreover, I feared for the health of the son's wife, a frail woman, who was at her husband's side so that she should not collapse. The hospital administration concurred with me. And so, the deceased stayed in her room, which was air-conditioned to prevent early decomposition. On the table near the bed, a candelabrum with two lights was burning. This had been the deceased's last act in life: lighting the (electric) Sabbath candlestick on the eve of the Sabbath.

Terminal Case – "Rabbi, What Is It Like to Die?"

A daughter asked me to speak to her mother, a terminal patient. The mother had the normal fear of death, and she asked, "How does it feel to die? What happens when one dies?" The daughter was in tears. In a calm and soothing manner, I replied to her, "Death is like falling asleep. Our soul returns to God, to our heavenly father. We return to our Heavenly Father. We are beyond pain."

Making the Morgue Area Respectable for Mourners

In the morgue waiting room we placed Hebrew and Hebrew-English books of Psalms as well as prayer books and yarmulkes for family members and shomrim (guardians who watch the body) to use for prayer. To help people who must spend many hours in that room, often during the Jewish Sabbath or a religious holiday, we placed a table, a few chairs, and a couch there. We also installed one of our Jewish chaplaincy's refrigerators. The waiting room has a sink and two washrooms. Posters requesting attention to keeping the area clean were hung on the walls.

May the All-Merciful One wipe away tears from all who suffer and have us serve Him in the paths of life.

14: HELPING NON-JEWISH PATIENTS

Visiting an Episcopal Pastor

I received a call from the chaplain of the Princeton Medical Center about an Episcopal patient of theirs who was transferred to our hospital. The chaplain requested that our Protestant chaplain visit with her. As we had no Protestant chaplain on our staff at that time, I was asked to see that patient, who appreciated my visits and my interest in her well-being. She underwent surgery on five strictures in the ileum, where, she said, the X-rays had not revealed any problem. I gave her support and comfort and also kept in touch with her Princeton chaplain, who had taken this lady's case to heart. When the chaplain and the lady's home church called regularly for information, I received ample thanks for my ministrations to this Episcopal patient.

"A Scholarly Question"

A non-Jewish staff member of our Medical Center left a message on my tape recorder, saying that she had "a scholarly question" for me. When I returned her call, she quoted the following Biblical verses to me, by heart and in English and asked if I could identify them: "For the land, whither thou goest in to possess it, is not like the land of Egypt, from whence ye came out, where thou didst sow thy seed and didst water it with thy foot, as a garden of herbs. But the land, whither ye go over to possess it, is a land of hills and valleys, and drinketh water of the rain of heaven." She thought they were somewhere in Isaiah. In fact, I told her, they are in Deuteronomy 11:10–11. I admired her exact English quote and complimented her on her knowledge. She is a young practicing Protestant, very much committed to religion and studying the Bible regularly.

From Distress to Joy

She was not of the Jewish faith, but her teacher at college, who had been a leader in a congregation I had served, had recommended that she contact me. I found her depressed and in tears. She said she had been very close to and also overprotected by her mother, who had passed on two months ago.

She had a happy marriage and two good children. Yet she felt unable to cope with life, and a physician had called her "a big baby," and that at age forty!

We discussed some of her rather immature attitudes and keen sensitivity, and her wish to continue college on a part-time basis in order to qualify as a kindergarten teacher. As she was just at the beginning of college, I suggested a more realistic solution of becoming a teacher's assistant. After an hour's session, she regained her composure as well as her self-confidence. When I saw her the next day she was out of bed and smiling, and she told me how much our session had helped her crystallize her thinking and open new vistas that were realistic and within her ability to cope with and find satisfaction. She bid me good-bye by kissing my hand.

Her husband called to tell me that he found that his wife began feeling better after my visit, for which he was most grateful, especially, as he put it, "since one does not find too many like you – people with a heart."

Non-Jewish Person Practicing Judaism

She had developed pneumonia and fever during her seventh month of pregnancy. Since her husband was Jewish, I found her name on the list of Jewish patients and visited her. She told me she had studied Judaism on her own for five years and was determined to undergo conversion. We discussed some of her problems about her life and her ideas, and she added that she was already practicing some of the observances of the Sabbath and *kashruth*. She loved Judaism and was so grateful for my clarifications.

Episcopal Patient Insists on Counseling by Rabbi

She called my office and requested my visit. She was an Episcopalian, but said she felt that her church devotes most of its time to helping the underprivileged in the world and, therefore, a rabbi would give her more personal attention and help her regain courage and perspective in life. She had come from out-of-town for treatment, and being alone with no close family anywhere, she wanted to move to New York, where positions had been offered to her by the United Nations and by Barnard College, of which she was an alumna. Above all, she needed to unburden herself and get reassurance and encouragement. I also guided her on ways to reorganize her life in this city. She was most grateful to me.

A Baptismal Certificate?

I found this young black man waiting for me at the door of my office. He had been directed to me. His request: a baptismal certificate from the chaplain who had baptized his infant son a few days earlier in our K9 neonatal ICU. He had not thought to get the name of the chaplain who did it and now wanted to get such a certificate from me – who certainly could not provide it. Upon reflection, it occurred to me that one of our Catholic chaplains might have performed this religious act. This certificate became so important to him because his child had died in another hospital, and the body remained in the morgue for two days because the family's parish church would not provide a religious service and burial until proof be brought that the infant had been baptized. My telephone call to Saint Cecilia's Rectory, where our Catholic chaplains resided, disclosed that they were on a retreat. Luckily, they provided me with a phone number in Rockland County, where I succeeded in getting in touch with the Catholic chaplain who had, indeed, performed the baptism. He consented to call the family's parish church, thereby resolving the sad problem that had been lingering with no solution in sight.

Learning from Rabbi's Report

An expression of gratitude from the Protestant chaplain at our hospital is among the scores included in my annual report describing how cases are handled by this rabbi and head chaplain. He revealed to us that he had shared our report with the Council of Churches, which had qualified it as "superb" and recommended reading subsequent reports for their educational and guidance values. We feel very gratified by the reception our writing has received and are glad to share our know-how with other interested personnel. Better service to patients and a measure of relief of human suffering and increased hope and peace of mind is likely to result.

Servicing Our Non-Jewish Patients

A staff of fifteen chaplains services the large number of our non-Jewish patients. I was particularly impressed with the numerous messages in my voice mail, as well as telephone calls, requesting ashes during Ash Wednesday. I passed the messages to the proper Christian clergymen. Indeed, religion plays a major role among our clientele and staff, and we are glad to be of service to all.

"Born Again Minister"

This patient called our office for a "born again minister." We never had such a request, and I know of no clergy classifying itself this way. Therefore, I suggested that she select a chaplain from our existing Christian staff. She selected a Protestant minister but insisted on getting the male chaplain rather than his associate, a lady minister, as, according to her, it did not "square with the Bible." Of course, we were glad to help this patient fulfill her religious needs her way. She appreciated our assistance.

Drawn to Judaism

A psychiatrist from our psychiatric ward called to request my visit with a patient who claimed she was interested in Judaism and wanted to see a rabbi. It turned out that, for psychological reasons, the patient refused to talk and communicated only by written messages on her pad and by gestures. She had been separated from her husband, who took their children, and was seeking a divorce from him. She expressed a strong interest in Judaism and attended our Sabbath services – all without talking. I saw her a few times at her request and at the request of her psychiatrist. She appreciated my visits but I could not get her to talk. I was surprised, therefore, when a few weeks after her discharge, she called for an appointment. She had somehow managed to establish contact with Orthodox rabbis on the West Side, where she lived, and also attended classes on Judaism given by a rabbi's wife. She revealed that she felt at peace only with Judaism. She also revealed that her father was a Greek Jew and that he and her natural mother, who was not Jewish, had abandoned her as a child. My counseling concentrated mainly on encouraging her to continue treatment as an outpatient, to try to resolve her marital problem and not to rush into conversion to Judaism as, according to Jewish teaching, she can attain salvation as a good and moral gentile. She continued to call on me and insisted on my accepting a skullcap and a wallet that she had made for me.

Non-Jew Asks for Rabbi's Prayer

She was not Jewish, but when I entered the semiprivate room and introduced myself to her Jewish roommate, she immediately came over to me. Her eyes full of tears, she asked me to offer a prayer for her mother, who had just died. I obliged and offered a prayer in English invoking God's solace to the soul of the deceased and Divine mercy and comfort to the distressed family. In this sad circumstance, it was my privilege to speak words that soothed the mind and brought relief to a suffering heart.

"Why Are You Crying?"

As I entered this room in the psychiatry ward, I noticed a young lady lying on her bed with tears rolling off her cheeks. I approached her, identified myself, and asked, "Why are you crying?"

In response, she asked me to close the door and, sitting up in her bed, said, "I love her more than him."

Not wanting to read more than its surface meaning into her statement, I replied, "You may love her as a friend but him you may come to regard as a potential spouse if you love him or find another man." We chatted for a while, and I encouraged her to talk this matter over freely with her physician. She also expressed her wish to go home. I reassured her that this was a short-term facility and that patients do get better here. "Give yourself a chance to recover health-wise and wait till the physician feels you are ready to be discharged."

She was not Jewish and knew my position. I briefed her on Catholic Mass at our hospital. My conversation with her brought her peace of mind and a smile to her face. She stretched out her arm to shake hands with me and reciprocated my parting words to her by saying, "God bless you, too."

"Please Say a Blessing on Me Too"

Often, the non-Jewish roommates of Jewish patients see me communicating with patients and ask, "Please say a blessing on me, too." I oblige, of course, and receive in turn a happy smile or a handshake.

Courtesy to Visiting Clergy

We had a problem in our psychiatry department when a visiting clergyman (not a hospital chaplain) was restricted to normal visiting hours and could not see a patient, a parishioner of his church, at the time he came. When apprised of this, I brought the case up for investigation and our correct policy was reaffirmed, namely, that visiting clergy can visit patients, including psychiatric patients, at any reasonable time at the clergyman's convenience. We are grateful to the director of Psychiatric Rehabilitation and Therapeutic Activities, a member of whose staff inadvertently caused the problem, for apologizing formally to the clergyman involved and again stressing our correct policy in this matter.

Introducing Catholic Patients to Catholic Chaplains

From time to time a Catholic patient would tell me that he had not received any visits from a chaplain of his faith. I must add that our Catholic chaplains are very conscientious and do an excellent job here. What probably occurred was that the name of the particular patient had not appeared on the census list under the code name C, which stands for Catholic, but was printed on a list without religious preference and the chaplain could not identify him as Catholic. In all such cases, I either give the patient the phone number of our priests or I make the call myself. Of course, I extend my good wishes to the patient and regularly receive a "Thank you very much, Rabbi," in response.

An Episcopalian Unburdens Himself

He had a Jewish-sounding name, and I visited him. He suffered from cancer and now expected surgery of bone in his chin. He was a singer, so this type of surgery upset him with unusual force. I listened sympathetically to his tale of woe and offered some words of hope. "I am fortunate to have [met] you," he added. "I am an Episcopalian and was raised as such. My grandfather, however, was Jewish. Thank you for coming to see me."

Child to Visit Infectious Mother

The patient's pastor called on me to obtain permission for a nine-year-old child to visit her infectious mother. He felt the child was getting disturbed by the mother's absence and feared she was dead. Usually such young children are not allowed to visit. As the pastor offered to have the child brought over by another minister in the absence of the father, I obtained permission for the visit, on the condition that the minister carefully supervise the child and not let her kiss the mother for fear of catching the disease.

Priestly Appreciation

In one of our ICUs, I found a Greek-Orthodox priest as a patient. I approached his bed, introduced myself, and asked if our regular Greek-Orthodox chaplain had visited him. The answer was affirmative. Still, he appreciated my interest and my good wishes to him, and kissed my hand as we parted.

Hanukkah in the Bible?

A Protestant minister called up to find information on the sources of Hanukkah in the Bible. Answer: The Books of the Maccabees are not included in the Hebrew Bible but belong to the Apocrypha literature. The story of the menorah is recorded in the Talmud.

Bless Me Too

As I visited a Jewish patient, I suddenly heard a voice from behind a curtain say, "Bless me too. I am going for surgery today." It was a non-Jewish patient's voice. I obliged, of course, and received many thanks in return.

Jewish Sounding Name

A non-Jewish patient with a Jewish sounding name was placed on my list. I visited her. Said she: "I am not Jewish but I expect you to visit me too when you visit my Jewish roommate." She felt strengthened by my visit.

Visiting a Lutheran Pastor

This Lutheran pastor came to our emergency unit and was diagnosed as needing an immediate appendectomy. A colleague of his called my office, requesting a chaplain's visit. I promised to make the visit myself and promptly – for which he was very grateful, and so was the patient. I visited him three times.

Non-Jewish Roommate Requests Our Prayer Texts

As I visited a Jewish patient and handed him some printed prayer texts, his non-Jewish roommate requested the same prayers. I obliged and received thanks in return.

Non-Jewish Family in Distress

They stood grave and saddened at the entrance to a room. I introduced myself and asked if I could be of some help. They said, "No, thank you." A few minutes later, they approached me in the hall and requested that I offer a prayer at the bedside of a terminal wife and mother. I obliged and recited a comforting Psalm in English. The family thanked me profusely.

Protestant Minister Asked Me to See a Child

A Protestant minister from New Jersey asked me to see a seven-year-old girl and her parents following the child's brain surgery at our hospital. The child was in surgery a long time. I later traced her to FICU, offered comfort to the distressed parents, had them see the child as she awakened, visited them a few days later, and offered emotional support.

15: UNIQUE SITUATIONS

Yiddish: Second Most Used Language Here

Besides English, the second most used language here among Jewish patients is Yiddish. Then come Hebrew, French, and German. It is usually our Hassidic patients, some Russian Jews, and some Holocaust survivors who communicate best in Yiddish. It is most helpful that I speak those five languages. They enable me to communicate directly with our patients and their families. I am also called by physicians and staff to translate from the patient's language to English.

Only French and Spanish – Good Enough!

I had the impression that she did not understand me, so I asked her what language she speaks. That she understood, and replied, "French and Spanish." Luckily, I managed to converse with her in French. She was a grand old lady from Paris and spoke a beautiful French which we both enjoyed. Yes, she also gratefully accepted my invitation to attend our hospital's Hanukkah celebration and concert.

"Just Spelling"

The nurse had a question: The family of a deceased patient asked her to write the name of the observance of the seven days of mourning. She just did not know how to spell the Hebrew word in English lettering, so she called. The spelling is: *SHIVAH*.

Interest in a Hebrew Song

I found a message from a non-Jewish hospital employee on my voice mail, asking me to identify and give her the full text of an Israeli song, part of which she sang into the phone. It began with the line "*Havah Nagilah*..." meaning "Let us be joyful" and is used mostly to welcome people at a function. She had heard that popular song in the past, and it appealed to her. I gave her the requested text. People naturally turn to the rabbi for information and explanation on whatever has to do with Jewish life.

Helping a Young Immigrant Find Job

A hospital staff member turned to me for help in locating a Jewish institution that would need a translator of religious material from English into Spanish. She needed it for a friend of hers who had emigrated from Argentina and works for the United Nations. However, volunteer work at a religious institution, she told me, would help that young lady in qualifying for residence here. Upon hearing this problem, it occurred to me that the Lubavitcher Hassidic movement, which issues religious material for many countries, might be just the right place for that young lady. Therefore, I made the contact, and I am glad to say that this "match" worked out very well for both parties.

Hebrew Marriage Document Translated into English

A psychologist turned to me with an unusual request. One of her clients did not have her civil marriage certificate, which was needed to entitle her to Medicaid. However, she did have her Jewish marriage document, called a ketubah. Therefore, I issued an English translation of the ketubah, with the pertinent information on the names of the couple and the date of the wedding in 1924, which I obtained by finding the civil date corresponding to the Hebrew date in a Hebrew-English calendar.

Two Teenagers Observe Our Emergency Department

I received a request from a prominent rabbi and educator to obtain permission for two high school students at an upstate yeshiva to spend sixteen hours of clinical observation in our Emergency Department. They needed it as part of their training as emergency medical technicians. Both boys wanted to come to the city on Thursday and stay for the weekend before returning to their school upstate. They wanted their training to take place in two stages: on Friday from 8:00 A.M. to 4:00 P.M. and on Saturday night from midnight to 8:00 A.M. I was glad to have obtained permission from the proper authorities at our hospital. Our emergency staff subsequently gave those students a very high rating.

Overflowing with Biblical and Talmudic Knowledge

This distinguished rabbinic personality enjoyed my frequent visits, during which his knowledge of Judaism flowed like a perennial spring. Like a fountain spouting water, so did his scholarship keep pouring out of his mind and heart. He had spent a lifetime in the rabbinate and had concentrated on learning during every free moment, day or night, so that he amassed a vast encyclopedic treasury of Bible and Talmud. These sessions added well-being to him.

His devoted wife and daughters and nurse were always with him, while other members of the family took turns spending time with him. When he laid down his burden of illness and returned his soul to his Maker, his grown daughters, mothers themselves, unabashedly shed tears. I offered words of solace to the family in their hour of grief. I told them that the rabbi had been a tremendous success as a father as well as a teacher.

Fear of Intruder

This elderly patient was all apprehensive about a telephone call he had received during his hospital stay, asking him details such as whether he lived in a private home or in an apartment building, and his exact address. Whereupon fear overtook him that a clever intruder might break into his apartment where his wife had remained alone. To reassure the patient, I called up our preadmission office, which confirmed that they had called the patient, who had been admitted through the Emergency Department without having filled out all the hospital forms. The patient relaxed, having regained his peace of mind.

A Preaching Roommate

This young mother from the Midwest was treated at our hospital with experimental drugs for a prolonged period of time. I had given her a great deal of guidance and comfort. Now she called, requesting an urgent visit. Her new roommate, of Hassidic inclination, tried to change her outlook and lifestyle through constant preaching, which was uncalled for as it increased guilt and lacked in tact. I told the young mother how to tell the preacher that she does not feel well and would appreciate her stopping the well-meaning lectures. Then I directly requested the roommate to desist, as her preaching only served to upset a very sick patient who needed all her strength and peace of mind to keep up with her treatment and overcome her loneliness, with her family being far away from New York. The roommate understood and desisted.

"Fantastic Accommodation"

This patient came all the way from the South to our oncology unit for a projected two-months' stay. His wife, who accompanied him, felt that she should assist him by being at his bedside all day long. She had a problem finding a room to rent for two months. I was able to locate such a place for her near the hospital, and she was treated like a member of the family there, with the added benefit of reasonable rent. Every time I visited this patient, he and his wife reiterated their appreciation for this help and added that it was a "fantastic accommodation."

Young Hassid – A Bone Marrow Donor for Unknown Recipient

I was called to the recovery room on Annenberg 6 to see a religious man who volunteered to be a bone marrow donor and asked that the rabbi see him. He turned out to be a recently married Hassidic man of twenty-two, with beard and sidelocks. He was uncomfortable, in pain and groggy, and still under the effects of the anesthesia. He was later transferred to a regular room, where his mother visited him. Although his vital signs were good, she was told he would have to spend the night at the hospital.

His mother told me that his bone marrow specimen was immediately flown to a twenty-eight-year-old mother whose marrow matched his. Indeed, I was highly impressed by this act of selfless sacrifice for a total stranger. He just wanted to give something of himself to an unknown needy person.

I called his deed an act of heroism and courage.

Question from an Outsider

An unknown physician from Saint John's Hospital in Queens called to ask me what to send Jewish mourners on the loss of a relative, a former patient in that hospital. Since they wanted something tangible, I recommended planting trees in Israel, which now costs $5.00 per tree. The Jewish National Fund issues special certificates inscribed with the donor's name as well as the name of the deceased in whose memory the gift is being made. I found it meaningful that many outsiders turn to us for guidance.

Iranian-Jewish Family Solicits Rabbi's Blessings

She and her two sisters took a taxi from Brooklyn to see me. I was of some help to her husband who had been a patient here, and, since that time, they have turned to me with their problems. They are Iranian Jews, whose custom it is to see a rabbi and ask for spiritual help. This time, they who were of childbearing age wanted me to give them special blessings that they should have children. Since prayer talks and wishes had helped the husband in his business enterprise, the two other sisters requested similar blessings for prosperity as well.

They had one more problem: there was a very gifted daughter of marriageable age who was finding it difficult to find a match, and they wanted my help in that, too. In addition to blessings for success, I gave them the telephone number of a marriage broker in a reputable Jewish organization. The needs of the people are many, says a Talmudic prayer. But for this Iranian-Jewish family, the way to success was clear.

Daytime Learning? Go to Patients' Library

A family member of a patient, a rabbinical student, inquired first about the location of the closest synagogue in order to attend services. I gave him the information. He then asked about a place where he could step in during the day and do some learning. I recommended our patients' library, where he could find a fair collection of religious books for study, such as the *Chumash* (Pentateuch) with *Mikraoth Gedoloth* (commentaries) and a complete set of the Talmud, which we purchased with the special Federation Fund allocated to our Jewish chaplaincy. That was just what he was seeking.

Making it Ethical

A family called to seek guidance for a patient who was urged to have extensive heart surgery. We advised them to get a second opinion from another physician, highly regarded in our hospital. It turned out that the family had already contacted that cardiologist who declined to come because it would not be ethical to interfere with another physician's case. Since a decision on surgery had to be made without much delay, I myself contacted the physician in charge of the case and had *him* call the consultant, who then agreed to come. This approach was helpful to all.

"Sympathy for Jews"

The patient's physician asked that I visit him. Though it turned out that he was not Jewish, he welcomed me heartily. He told me he had no religion and that his parents were not Jewish. Still, he added, "I feel sympathy for the Jews, and I feel more Jewish than anything else." We chatted for a long while, and he was very grateful that a rabbi had visited him.

Being Observed by a Supreme Court Judge

One gets a special lift when one receives a letter from an unexpected source that, unbeknown to us, had been observing our work. An acting justice of the Supreme Court of New York wrote, in part: "In your role at Mount Sinai, you have been a model leader. You do make a difference at Sinai, and I hope God will bless you with health and joy always."

Obtaining Scholarship for Employee's Son

A Russian-Jewish woman, a hospital employee, wanted assistance in having her young son admitted not only to yeshiva, but to a yeshiva of her choice that has difficult admission requirements, and she requested a scholarship! I was able to fulfill her desire.

Emergency Room Call and Isaiah 58

As soon as I arrived at my office in the morning, the Patient Representative office called and asked for my urgent visit to the emergency department. It turned out that an elderly Jewish lady had been brought there in the middle of the night, and the staff did not know how to help her. As I conversed with her in both Yiddish and English, it became clear that she was starved, and that she wanted to be admitted to our hospital as a regular patient. She suffered from bronchitis, which, our staff asserted, does not require hospitalization, and, therefore, they suggested that she go home. However, being completely alone and paralyzed on the left side following a stroke, she begged us to allow her to stay until she recovered from the bronchitis and coughing which caused her much pain.

I had a kosher breakfast brought to her but she could not handle it with the use of only one hand. I then fed this starved elderly lady while the message of the prophet Isaiah (chapter 58) ran through my mind. It is chanted in the synagogue on Yom Kippur and admonishes us to offer bread to the hungry and feed the famished person. With this religious view in mind, I felt it is not below rabbinic dignity to literally feed the hungry.

Following calls to the lady's private physician in Brooklyn, and after soliciting the help of the doctors in Emergency, a thorough physical examination ensued. After additional calls to her doctor, who suggested having her transferred by ambulance to a hospital with which he was affiliated, the problem was resolved when her private physician arrived. I had spent three hours on this case, which was ultimately resolved in a humane way.

"Please See Me. I Am in Mythology. . ."

It was a late winter afternoon, about an hour before sunset. My voice mail had a message for me, but all I could make out was that the man wanted phylacteries (tefillin) in order to pray before sunset. His name was not given. He only said, "You know me." His location came out in a blurred fashion: "I am in...Mythology," followed by "Annenberg 3." Obviously the man had had no chance to pray the morning service with phylacteries and wanted to do so before the day was gone. Whereupon I strolled through Annenberg 3 to look for a Hassidic person who could have left that message for me. I had covered the complete floor when I suddenly saw a bearded old man in Hematology. I approached him and confirmed that he was the one who had left the message. He was sitting next to his daughter, who had brought him to our hospital and was preparing a Hebrew lesson plan for her teaching job. They were both very happy to see me. I took him to an unoccupied room and helped him put on the phylacteries that I had brought for him. He told me that today was the first time in his life that he was unable to pray with phylacteries in the morning, and he was so grateful that I had helped him keep a straight record. I was glad for him and glad to have found him – even not in Mythology but in Hematology!

Unlisted Patient Is Put in Contact with Chaplain of His/Her Faith

Each patient follows the In-patient Bed Census List arranged according to religion. If, at times, a patient turns out not to be Jewish or is unlisted, I ask whether a priest or minister has visited them or whether they would like such a visit. I then pass their names and room numbers to the proper Christian chaplain. All our chaplains thus cooperate in informing the correct chaplain for the patient. Our patients are very grateful for this service.

16: AFTERWORD BY FELLOW CLERGY AND OTHERS

I just read your report distributed by Mount Sinai at your initiative. What you are doing is nothing less than a *Kiddush Hashem* and an inspiration to the entire community.

– Dr. Norman Lamm, President,
Yeshiva University

After a long and very distinguished tenure as chaplain, you certainly deserve the independence and opportunity to pursue the many avenues in scholarship and travel that may have been long delayed because of your absolutely dedicated and inspired service to the sick and their families which was your hallowed charge. On the other hand, I know that the hospital and the patients of the future will sorely miss the ministrations that were distinctly yours. We at Yeshiva have always taken much pride in your illustrious career as rabbi and chaplain.

– Rabbi Zevulun Charlop, Dean,
Rabbi Isaac Elchanan Theological Seminary
Yeshiva University

Your activities are certainly inspiring, and the impact you have made is impressive. The Jewish community is, indeed, blessed to have someone of your stature and character serve the needs of so many different people on different levels.

– Rabbi Robert S. Hirt, Vice President for
Administration and Professional Education
Yeshiva University

All of those who ever came in contact with you in your capacity as head chaplain have sung your praises. Your sincerity and purpose, your devotion to the needs of patients, your desire to enhance Jewish life and tradition within The Mount Sinai Medical Center are all attributes which have brought about successes hitherto unknown within that institution. You performed an invaluable service in a way that is a *Kiddush Hashem*

Berabim! I do hope you reap a measure of the great satisfaction you obviously brought to others."

– Dr. Herbert C. Dobrinsky,
Vice President for University Affairs
Yeshiva University

In all my experience, I have never seen a more dedicated and devoted chaplain, one who has done far beyond the call of duty for the sake of the patients, their emotional, spiritual, and physical well being, and for the sake of Heaven. Your work is a true *Kiddush Hashem*.

– Rabbi Dr. Nisson Shulman,
Director, Rabbinic Placement
Yeshiva University

Thank you so much for your copy of your annual report. I look forward to receiving it yearly, so I can continue to marvel at the *Kiddush Hashem* which you render on a daily basis. Continued *Bracha* and *Hatzlacha*.

– Rabbi Steven M. Dworkin,
Executive Vice President,
Rabbinical Council of America

All of us know what a wonderful job you did at Mount Sinai and how much of yourself you invested in building a wonderful chaplaincy. You have brought honor to yourself, the chaplaincy, and the New York Board of Rabbis, and I am confident that hundreds, even thousands, of patients and staff members look to you in gratitude and with affection. Enjoy your retirement and your visit to Israel, and be assured that you go forward to the future with all of our blessings always.

– Rabbi Gilbert S. Rosenthal
Executive Vice President
New York Board of Rabbis

It is clear that you do so much for your large and diverse community, taking into account the special needs of various groups. Your dedication and caring are evident in all you do, as you bring relief and comfort to patients and their families. How wonderful that your work serves as a model for other chaplaincy programs, and that others learn from your personal and professional example.

– Rabbi Levi Meier, Ph.D., Chaplain,
Cedars-Sinai Medical Center
Los Angeles, California

I am amazed at the enormous changes in Mt. Sinai. The range of your activities is wide and has substantial depth. By continuing with your marvelous work, you have created a *Kiddush Hashem*.

– Rabbi Albert B. Schwartz, Director, Chaplaincy Commission, Fort Lauderdale, Florida

You are, of course, excellent in instilling hope and confidence in those patients who need, often desperately, your counsel and guidance. You are doing splendid work! We need more in this world who, like you, really want to help others.

– Dr. Otis E. Fellows,
Professor of French Literature,
Columbia University

His appointment as head chaplain at Mount Sinai offered him a splendid opportunity to combine his profound religious commitment and his exceptional sensitivity in counseling and assisting countless patients and their loved ones with compassion, understanding, and dedication. He has given of himself day and night, weekdays as well as weekends. He offers spiritual comfort at the bedside of patients and sees to it that special religious needs are met. His record of accomplishments at Mount Sinai commands awe and respect. The scope, quality, and effectiveness of Rabbi Spirn's activities as head chaplain serve as a model for hospitals everywhere.

– Dr. Benjamin J. Klebaner,
Professor of Economics,
City College of CUNY

Having been on the staff here at Mt. Sinai in the capacity of Catholic chaplain, I have come to know and admire Rabbi Spirn. He was most effective in my own orientation and understanding of the chaplaincy work here at Mt. Sinai. He has maintained a most inviting open door policy to his office and has been unequivocal in his insights to the work we carry out each day. He exemplifies diligence and is extremely conscientious in his chaplaincy care. He is always eager to listen and lend a helping hand. His work schedule is matched only by his thoroughness in seeing that all tasks and requests are carried out to the smallest detail. Perhaps I may conclude with paraphrasing some words of William Shakespeare and apply them to Rabbi Spirn, "His life is gentle and the elements so mixed in him that all creation might stand up and say – this is a man," – and truly, a man of God.

– Rev. George E. Baker, Catholic chaplain

I have known Rabbi Spirn since his arrival at the Mount Sinai Medical Center – 1979. During these years, he has been more than a rabbi and a chaplain. He has been a colleague. He has worked with me in the care and management of patients with their problems. His attentiveness to patients is exemplary. He responds almost immediately to patients with questions and problems. His sensitivity adds greatly to the actual medical care of the patients. His leadership sparked the formation of the kosher kitchen and cafeteria and the Peck Jewish Chapel. Both of these installations have added immeasurably to the comfort of Jewish patients and have enhanced the reputation of the Medical Center. He has introduced for the staff adult education programs for the study of Hebrew and the understanding of Jewish prayer. In addition to conducting the Sabbath and holiday services, he conducts magnificent celebrations of Passover and Hanukkah. One has to be inspired to attend these occasions and watch patients, doctors, nurses, attendants, enjoy themselves as they understand these holidays. There is absolutely no doubt that Rabbi Spirn's performance and activities are superior. His colleagues will unanimously attest to this appraisal.

– Dr. Donald Gribetz, Professor of Pediatrics

Conclusion by Rabbi Spirn:

I find the reciprocated warmth with which patients, staff, and colleagues view me as particularly meaningful. I felt gratified giving insightful pastoral and religious support to patients and to respond to physicians' requests for assistance in special cases. That Jewish patients and staff asked me questions on religion was natural. However, non-Jewish staff too turned to me frequently with questions about Judaism, which helped them in their care of Jewish patients. During the High Holy Day season, in particular, I was deeply touched by the good wishes so many extended to me as they saw me making my rounds in our institution. Somehow, it was as if I personified the Jewish faith here. It was a big responsibility but also an honor and a source of satisfaction which I carry with me as I retire after twenty-eight years as a community rabbi and close to twenty years as head chaplain at Mount Sinai.

APPENDIX

PROPOSAL FOR A KOSHER KITCHEN AT THE MOUNT SINAI MEDICAL CENTER

by
RABBI DR. CHARLES A. SPIRN, HEAD CHAPLAIN

I. Historic Background

When we were first established in 1852 as Jews' Hospital, we were completely kosher. In fact, as I read the archives of those early years, I was profoundly impressed by our founding fathers' commitment to fundamental Jewish principles as expressed in their constitution and in their deeds. When problems presented themselves, the leadership had recourse to Chief Rabbi Adler of London, England, and his decisions on Jewish law (halakhah) were gratefully accepted as binding. In 1866, the institution's name was changed to The Mount Sinai Hospital. The exact date when our hospital ceased to be kosher is an enigma. A noted American-Jewish historian whom I consulted thinks it happened soon after the change in name. Be that as it may, the fact remains that, at present, 40 percent of our patients are Jewish and among them, as will be shown later in this proposal, a sizable proportion (20 percent) abides by the kosher code of the Bible on principle as does also a sizable number of staff. It is primarily for the patients and, in addition, for staff that the introduction of an auxiliary kosher kitchen is an urgent need.

II. Statement of Objectives

In writing this proposal, I follow in the main the outline of a questionnaire submitted to me by Mr. Steph Slater, acting associate director of Support Services.

A. Commitment to the Jewish Community

Our hospital's "Strategic Guidelines for Patient Care Services" clearly and naturally admits our special commitment to the Jewish community. It states that "Mount Sinai will maintain its special relationship with the Jewish population." Obviously, that relationship cannot mean giving the Jewish patient better medical treatment, for that would be contrary to Jewish ethics and general American and medical practice. It must therefore refer to areas of special concern to Jews qua Jews. The observance of the Jewish dietary laws is such a major area for it requires much special consideration as well as sympathetic understanding of the religious sensitivities of those who abide by said laws. Furthermore, the organized Jewish community has in fact expressed itself openly on this point. Thus, Federation of Jewish Philanthropies (through its Religious Department), the New York Board of Rabbis (over the signatures of its Orthodox, Conservative, and Reform officers and its executive director) and the Rabbinical Council of America (Modern Orthodox) have all urged our hospital in writing to open a kosher kitchen. The Jewish religious community stands thus united in petitioning us to meet this fundamental Jewish religious need.

B.Commitment to Jewish Patients and Staff

Article V of the Mission Statement of The Mount Sinai Medical Center reads: "Mount Sinai will be ever sensitive to the social and health care needs of the many different communities it serves. The Center will be a participant in efforts to define and solve health problems in population groups and communities." Food certainly is a health problem and a daily necessity. A study of our menus reveals that the general community of patients at our hospital has been provided daily with quality food choices, including bacon, ham, salt pork, lobster, oysters, shrimp, etc. – all foods not acceptable to the Jewish kosher patients. I propose equality of treatment and more of a Jewish image of our hospital vis-à-vis the American-Jewish community.

C.Scope of Proposed Service

While I would applaud the idea of a completely kosher hospital similar to what we were once and to the present five hospitals in Metropolitan New York (Beth Israel, Albert Einstein, Brookdale, Kingsbrook Jewish, Maimonides), I will be satisfied with an auxiliary kosher kitchen for all patients who request it and for all staff members who want to buy a kosher meal during their working day at our Medical Center.

III.Present Kosher Meals Accommodations

A.Meals Served to Patients and Staff

...Our kosher patients are given presently TV dinners that come to the hospital in a packaged frozen state and are unfrozen and heated here. Patients react adversely to them. This led our Nutrition Office to keep on changing companies producing kosher dinners – we now purchase from four companies – with very little marked improvement in quality. Writes Mrs. Linda Lawson, our executive dietician, and Ms. Anne Cornfield, her assistant: "The quality of the kosher food is substandard." Our patients want freshly cooked tasty meals.

...The Satmar Hassidic group, unsatisfied with our food services but fully confident in our medical services, comes twice daily with mini buses from Williamsburgh and brings homemade meals to members of their group at the hospital. They have also responded positively to my appeals for food for non-Satmar patients who, out of desperation, ask me to get them kosher food from any outside source. And so we have the daily sight of Hassidic and other religious people coming to our hospital carrying containers of food for patients who cannot eat our food while their bills include payment for food not taken.

...Fluid diets, prescribed by physicians, are not available most of the time (examples: kosher bouillon, kosher jelly, etc.), with the result that we get the patients upset and affect adversely their medical treatment.

- Our personnel unwittingly compound the problem by adding nonkosher sausage on trays or mixing meat with milk and butter.
- Our kosher eating staff brings its food from home every day, and our kosher medical students have problems with preparing lunch and resort to the TV dinners for supper while bemoaning to the rabbi the absence of proper food.

B.Cost of Present Services

Mr. Sunder Raj, food services comptroller, responding to my inquiry, gave me the cost of food alone. He writes. "In 1981, we have purchased $98,750 worth of kosher food for patients." The Saga Corporation, which has made a study of our food services and has submitted its estimate for a kosher kitchen as well (page 78), gives us a figure close to that of Mr. Raj and adds more facts: "Present cost is $101,287 for packs plus $1.64/meal for base charge = $89,790. Total present cost is $191,077."

C.Evaluation of Need by Our Staff

Here are a few testimonies by our staff as made at our Food Services Evaluation Committee study sessions:

- *Mrs. Linda Lawson, executive dietician, and Ms. Anne Cornfield, assistant*: "The accommodation of our kosher patients is below optimum levels. Many times, the kosher packs are not ready on time or were *never* received in the house or the correct kosher pack is not given to the patient or the quality of the food is substandard."

- *Mrs. Ruth Ravich, patient representative:* "Kosher food is always a problem.
- *Mrs. Carol Nicol, associate director, Nursing Administration:* "Kosher food is a monumental difficulty."
- *Rabbi Spirn, head chaplain, in daily contact with Jewish patients:* "There is a crying need for a kosher kitchen. Its time has come now."

These testimonies corroborate the steady flow of numerous verbal and written complaints received by our hospital from patients on this subject. It is a daily persistent problem that just cannot be wished away but has to be faced and resolved.

IV.Market Demand

I have made a study of the market demand for a kosher kitchen at our hospital. Here are the results:

A.Patients

This past January, I obtained from Mrs. Lawson lists of the kosher pack tally sheet which indicates the patient's pavilion and bed number and what he/she ordered for lunch and dinner. Since many kosher patients order both meals, I have crossed out the double listing of a patient so as to get the number of kosher patients per day rather than the number of meals.

Result: Our kitchen served *between* 65 *and* 69 kosher patients daily.

In addition, the Satmar Hassidic group that I consulted told me they bring to our hospital meals for 18 *to* 20 patients daily.

Total daily kosher patients: 83 to 89

B.Staff

A poll taken by me of staff members who would use our kosher kitchen yielded 150 *names* and my study of kosher abiding staff is not complete. My lists comprise staff in practically every department in our hospital: from physicians, faculty, residents, students, to administration, engineering, records, social work, nursing, etc.

C.Visitors

Specifically families of patients that spend the major part of the day near their sick ones. They would appreciate a good, warm, kosher meal.

Suggestion – Our kosher kitchen should be equipped to handle 200 to 250 persons.

D. Comparison

For comparison's sake, it will be enlightening to know that hospitals with less of a kosher market than ours did feel the responsibility to install auxiliary kitchens on their premises. Here are a few names and figures that we have obtained:

Menorah Medical Center in Kansas City, Missouri: 16 kosher patients
Long Island Jewish Hospital: 27 kosher patients
Cedars-Sinai in Los Angeles, California: 41 kosher patients
Sinai Hospital in Baltimore, Md.: 69 kosher patients
Mount Sinai Hospital in Cleveland, Ohio: 90 kosher patients

VIII. Conclusion

In a formal letter to me dated October 11, 1979, and confirming my appointment as head chaplain of The Mount Sinai Hospital, Mr. Samuel Davis, director and now president, writes in part: "I am looking forward to the development of a program of religious support for the patients and their staff under your leadership." My annual report gives a comprehensive view of all my activities at our hospital and my responses to challenges in ways that alleviate human suffering and strengthen patients and staff spiritually and psychologically. Whatever depends on my efforts and abilities is carried out unobtrusively and efficiently. The kosher kitchen, however, is one project for which I must solicit the understanding heart and the helping hand of the top leadership of this our hospital. Its need is obvious and is being expressed all too frequently by patients of ours in whose well-being we have a stake. In this proposal, I am their spokesman. The expense for a kosher kitchen will be modest in our total eight million dollars food service budget, and some expense for food is part of what every patient pays for and is automatically entitled to. I predict that a kosher kitchen will be a huge success. Moreover, it will promote the raising of funds from the religious community. It will also be a big step in recognition of and loyalty to our early founders who had created a kosher hospital. And last but not least, it will add honor and prestige to The Mount Sinai Medical Center as the flagship of Jewish-sponsored hospitals in the world.

April 1982

The Board of Trustees accepted this Proposal and installed a kosher kitchen and cafeteria at The Mount Sinai Medical Center.